AF740536

# How to Teach the Epidural Block in Obstetric Anesthesia

Giorgio Capogna
Editor

# How to Teach the Epidural Block in Obstetric Anesthesia

Springer

*Editor*
Giorgio Capogna
EESOA European School of Obstetric Anesthesia
Rome, Italy

ISBN 978-3-031-70210-5 ISBN 978-3-031-70211-2 (eBook)
https://doi.org/10.1007/978-3-031-70211-2

The original submitted manuscript has been translated into English. The translation was done using artificial intelligence. A subsequent revision was performed by the author(s) to further refine the work and to ensure that the translation is appropriate concerning content and scientific correctness. It may, however, read stylistically different from a conventional translation.

© The Editor(s) (if applicable) and The Author(s), under exclusive license to Springer Nature Switzerland AG 2024
This work is subject to copyright. All rights are solely and exclusively licensed by the Publisher, whether the whole or part of the material is concerned, specifically the rights of translation, reprinting, reuse of illustrations, recitation, broadcasting, reproduction on microfilms or in any other physical way, and transmission or information storage and retrieval, electronic adaptation, computer software, or by similar or dissimilar methodology now known or hereafter developed.
The use of general descriptive names, registered names, trademarks, service marks, etc. in this publication does not imply, even in the absence of a specific statement, that such names are exempt from the relevant protective laws and regulations and therefore free for general use.
The publisher, the authors and the editors are safe to assume that the advice and information in this book are believed to be true and accurate at the date of publication. Neither the publisher nor the authors or the editors give a warranty, expressed or implied, with respect to the material contained herein or for any errors or omissions that may have been made. The publisher remains neutral with regard to jurisdictional claims in published maps and institutional affiliations.

This Springer imprint is published by the registered company Springer Nature Switzerland AG
The registered company address is: Gewerbestrasse 11, 6330 Cham, Switzerland

If disposing of this product, please recycle the paper.

# Preface

*To all my students who have become teachers*

Essentially, we teach as we were taught, when we first learned by watching and then directly on the patient, with the help of a tutor. Even today, the typical teaching of epidural catheter placement in obstetric anesthesia (as well as in other surgical and pain therapy settings) consists of a mix of theoretical didactic training and practical experience, in which the student and teacher together face the task in a clinical setting, using the patient as a learning model.

Teaching method is not usually standardized, is hardly formalized and institutionalized, and is highly variable among different university institutes, even in the same country.

Epidural block is indeed a complex procedure and requires cognitive skills such as the knowledge of the anatomy and of the procedure along with psychomotor skills such as the skills required to perform the technique. Therefore, it is commonly believed that training in epidural technique concerns exclusively technical aspects and, subsequently, pharmacological aspects and how to deal with difficult cases or the treatment of possible complications. However, the success of the technique often also depends on the organizational and interdisciplinary communication skills of the anesthesiologist (nontechnical skills). It is therefore essential, from the very beginning of practical training on the patient, that the teacher also takes care of the "relational aspects" of the epidural block.

It is certainly difficult to train for technical aspects as well as for teamwork in relation to the insertion of an epidural catheter for labor analgesia in a clinical context. The laboring woman is suffering, the atmosphere can be tense, and training for teamwork along with technical skills in this situation may not be acceptable to the laboring woman.

For this reason, a well-structured teaching method and simulation can provide a safe learning environment where patients are not exposed or harmed and, moreover, offers the possibility of practicing repetitively.

With this book, we aim to fill the gaps due to the absence of similar books devoted exclusively to how to teach the epidural block and, specifically, how to teach it in obstetrics.

We hope that this text will contribute to the creation of a structured, routinely applied, shared, validated, and controlled teaching method in every university or teaching institution entrusted with the preparation of future obstetric anesthesiologists.

*Please note that, due to the international readership of this book, in the text the terms "student," "resident," and "trainee" are indifferently used to define the "physician-in-training who is learning the epidural technique."*

Rome, Italy Giorgio Capogna

# Contents

# Contributors

**Emanuele Capogna** European School of Obstetric Anesthesia, Maternal and Neonatal Simulation Center EESOA, Rome, Italy

**Giorgio Capogna** EESOA European School of Obstetric Anesthesia, Rome, Italy

**Gian Luigi Gonnella** Institute of Anesthesiology and Intensive Care Medicine, Sacro Cuore Catholic University, Rome, Italy

**Ilaria Pacini** Department of Anesthesiology, IRCSS Istituto Ortopedico Rizzoli, Bologna, Italy

**Marco Scorzoni** Institute of Anesthesiology and Intensive Care Medicine, Sacro Cuore Catholic University, Rome, Italy

# Teaching the Epidural Technique

Giorgio Capogna

Even today, the teaching of the epidural technique often takes place in the field where the trainee and the teacher face the technique together on the patient, who is used as a learning model. The teaching method is not usually standardized and varies greatly among different university institutes. In this chapter, the general principles of teaching and learning will be illustrated.

## 1 Introduction

"The student and the teacher scrub themselves, put on sterile gloves, and together face the first epidural puncture. The former performs all the preliminary maneuvers, chooses the suitable interspinous space, and infiltrates the skin and deep tissues with local anesthetic; then, inserts the epidural needle to a depth of about 2 cm, while the teacher checks its orientation. From this moment on, the tasks are divided: the teacher grasps the needle and advances it, while the student exerts trembling compressive movements on the piston of the syringe filled with air until the epidural space is reached. At this point, the teacher also checks the loss of resistance and, if satisfied with the placement of the needle, entrusts the student with the subsequent tasks of inserting the catheter, removing the needle, and performing an aspiration test through the catheter, carefully supervising him. When the teacher believes that the student has acquired a good sensitivity regarding the decrease in resistance, the roles are reversed: the student will insert the needle and the teacher will compress the piston of the syringe. Finally, the student is allowed to do everything on his own, while the teacher, washed and with sterile gloves on, observes, ready to correct any mistakes, if necessary." These are the words with which, in 1978, our great master

G. Capogna (✉)
EESOA European School of Obstetric Anesthesia, Rome, Italy
e-mail: capogna.eesoa@gmail.com

© The Author(s), under exclusive license to Springer Nature Switzerland AG 2024
G. Capogna (ed.), *How to Teach the Epidural Block in Obstetric Anesthesia*,
https://doi.org/10.1007/978-3-031-70211-2_1

Philip Bromage described in his book *Epidural Analgesia* [1] how to teach the epidural technique.

It is curious to note that Prof. Bromage, despite describing and recommending the technique of loss of resistance to saline, then used the air when describing the stages of teaching the technique. Another thing to note is how, more than 40 years ago, Bromage deprecated the method of having the student practice the epidural technique without having previously used what he called "auxiliary teaching means," which at the time were visual aids (slides, videotapes, films) and tactile methods (anatomical dissection, artificial models).

His chapter on the teaching technique begins like this: "Good manual skills in performing puncture and epidural analgesia are not difficult to learn. As with all other manual skills, they must be well taught to prevent the learner from acquiring bad habits, but at the same time, the patient must also be protected from the beginner during his educational process. In the past, instruction of this kind had always taken place according to a traditional pattern, with periods of apprenticeship. The beginner prepared himself alone, with appropriate introductory and propaedeutic readings, and then, together with the master, devoted himself to perfecting the clinical part, using patients (alive!) as models. This method led, inevitably, to a certain increase in accidental dural punctures and any consequent suffering on the part of the patient had to be accepted as an unpleasant but inevitable part of a teaching system, necessary for the ultimate care of the patient himself. Today, between the beginner and the patient, a number of simulator models can be placed, and before the beginner can even touch a living model, he must have acquired a considerable degree of manual skill. As a result, the number of dural punctures by trainees has significantly decreased" [1].

## 2 We Teach as We Were Taught

Essentially, we teach as we were taught, when we first learned by watching and then directly on the patient, with the help of a tutor. Even today, the typical teaching of epidural catheter placement in obstetric anesthesia (as well as in other surgical and pain therapy settings) consists of a mix of theoretical didactic training and practical experience, in which the student and teacher together face the task in a clinical setting, using the patient as a learning model.

This teaching method is not usually standardized, is hardly formalized and institutionalized, and is highly variable among different University Institutes.

Although anesthesia societies have issued some guidelines regarding the training of residents, teaching strategies are not clearly recommended or identified, and the guidelines themselves recognize that there is extreme diversity and disparity among different countries and, within the same country, among various institutes and specialization schools [2].

Both in Italy and in Europe, in some institutes, only residents who are not beginners or who are not in their first years of specialization and/or who have had previous experience with neuraxial blocks in other types of surgery (usually orthopedics) are admitted to obstetric anesthesia, but this does not guarantee that they have had previous experiences with epidural blocks, as the most common neuraxial practice in nonobstetric surgeries is spinal anesthesia. In some cases, only residents who have already performed a minimum number of spinal anesthetics are allowed to attend the delivery room, while in others, this requirement is not essential.

Generally, if the resident is an absolute beginner, he is allowed to observe for a certain period of time and then gradually try the technique in an assisted manner.

Usually, the didactic approach is very practical and directly *hands-on* and is not always preceded by formal classroom lessons on anatomy, technique, and materials.

In the absence of formal classroom lessons, scheduled by the training curriculum of the specialization school, the basic information necessary and preparatory to performing an epidural block is transmitted in various ways, from reading and personal study to the distribution of handouts, to participation in department meetings, and, in some cases, to self-learning uncontrolled by teachers.

The material for performing the block is presented in a highly variable manner, as it is the time dedicated to this educational session. Sometimes, the residents begin to learn about the materials at the same time as they perform the block for the first time.

The teaching technique used on the patient is highly variable and tutor-dependent, but generally, the process follows one or more of these steps (not necessarily in this chronological order):

The resident observes the block performed by the tutor without scrubbing and putting on sterile gloves.

The resident is instructed on the basic elements that precede the block: how to scrub in a sterile manner, how to put on gloves, how to position the patient, etc.

The resident observes the block performed by the tutor after learning to scrub and put on sterile gloves.

The resident tries to perform the block by placing his hands on those of the tutor (usually on the syringe plunger).

The resident tries to perform local anesthesia and/or insert the needle or start the procedure, which is then completed by the tutor.

The tutor starts the procedure (e.g., inserts the needle) which is then completed by the resident.

The resident tries to perform the block alone, but with the tutor also washed and ready to intervene and correct.

In some institutions, the resident performs the block "simultaneously and together" with the tutor.

The number of epidurals needed for the transition to the next step is generally tutor-dependent. Also, the number of epidurals assisted by the tutor (performed together) before the student can be left alone is highly variable and based more on local practice or the personal decision of the tutor, rather than being established by independent assessment methods (checklists, rating scales, and learning curves).

Tutors are generally present in the delivery room during the initial training period.

A formal institutional program reserved for tutors on how to teach epidurals or how to evaluate a student is very rare, even though the guidelines of the European Board of Anesthesia of the UEMS (EBA-UEMS) recommend the implementation of courses on "how to teach" [3].

Although there is widespread awareness that it would be appropriate for beginners not to learn directly on the patient immediately, but to follow a more articulated path that includes a more comprehensive evaluative approach, also and above all to reduce the number of errors and their potential effects on the patients themselves [4–6], the use of an epidural simulator is not yet routine nor standardized as a mandatory tool for the transition between theoretical lessons and practice on the patient.

When a simulator is used, the training technique is also highly variable. It can range from the use of a spine model to a commercial mannequin epidural simulator, or more rarely a haptic, or occasionally, a custom-built simulator can be used.

Even when the epidural simulator is used, the simulator exercise methodology is generally left to the experience or improvisation (of common sense) of individual tutors who generally do not follow any "instructions for use."

## 3 The Needs of the Students and Their Difficulties

A student's needs depend fundamentally on their previous experience and their knowledge base. A very simple way to assess a learner's needs is to ask them what they would like to "learn" that day: "Is there a particular topic you would like to discuss?" The purpose of this question is to find out what the student feels they need to learn. Motivations can obviously vary: the question may arise because the student has to take an exam soon or, more frequently, it is an unresolved issue or not sufficiently clarified from a previous clinical experience.

Being specific about learning needs can be difficult, and certainly, each teacher has their own effective way of proceeding on how to relate to the student, but in all cases, given an arbitrarily selected topic, it may be useful to discuss:

- What the student already knows and what they still cannot do and any previous unsuccessful attempts.
- What feedback they have received previously.
- What additional knowledge and skills may be needed to complete the case independently.
- Some examples of constructive phrases could be:
- If this were your case, what would prevent you from acting independently?
- What elements and advice/help do you need to move forward?
- How detailed do you want me to be?

These questions can help the student and the teacher identify aspects of a clinical case to focus on and highlight knowledge or skill gaps that deserve further discussion or that require additional practice.

Unfortunately, there are not many studies examining the opinions of students on the training received. In an Australian survey [7], all the trainees interviewed reported having received training based on practice guided by older colleagues. Complementary educational activities were not routinely offered but were available in varying percentages. For example, an introductory visit to the delivery room was reported in 56% of cases, a formal lesson in 56%, and practice on a simulator in only 13%. Competence was assessed variably but without any structured tool, nor were periodic evaluation meetings conducted. This study advocates the use of departmental audits to assess the learning progress of young anesthesiologists and, in particular, considers the first 20 epidurals as the critical moment to identify those who are developing their skills too slowly and therefore should be more supported. It is interesting to note that in this study, especially during the execution of the first epidurals, as many as 67% of the trainees reported that "performing an epidural was stressful" and that the same type of stress was reported in a quarter of the 200 trainees in another English survey [8], who in particular complained about the excessive environmental pressure exerted by midwives or other department staff.

Among other data, it should be noted that between 80 and 90% of respondents considered the number of cases in which they were trained with the help of a tutor before being left alone to be sufficient, and the same percentage believed they had received adequate explanation of spinal anatomy and the risks and complications of the technique. However, only half of the respondents believed they had the ability to solve technical difficulties on their own if they arose. In fact, 37% of respondents to the questionnaire reported having had an accidental dural puncture during the execution of their first 25 epidurals.

In accordance with the more than 30-year teaching experience of the author of this book, also confirmed by a more recent (unpublished) survey from the Catholic University of Rome, based on informal open-ended interviews, the main training objectives expressed by trainees starting their internship in the delivery room were (in order of importance and frequency of response):

The ability to perform an epidural autonomously without the presence of a tutor.
The ability to solve problems that arise during the technical execution of the block.
The ability to deal with any complications.
Acquiring theoretical knowledge of anatomy and technique.

The main basic difficulties encountered by beginners in the epidural procedure include:

(a) How to identify the interspace and orient the needle with the desired angle, so that no contact with the bone occurs.
(b) How to identify false or pseudo loss of resistance. In some institutions, when teaching the epidural block, the needle is inserted a few centimeters into the soft tissues and not on the dorsal aspect of the ligamentum flavum, for fear of accidentally perforating the dura and to put the trainee at ease. In this way, the needle may be located between the soft tissues, well before the epidural space,

and if the loss of resistance procedure with a syringe is started at this stage, it can give rise to a false loss of resistance.

(c) How to recognize the type of bone contact and how to correctly redirect the needle on the right path based on the angle of inclination of the needle, its depth, the position of the vertebrae, and the tactile sensations returned by the needle itself.

(d) Being able to position the needle within the epidural space in such a way that it protrudes as little as possible, in order to minimize the risk of puncturing the dura. The protrusion of the epidural needle is defined as the distance between the tip of the needle that has just passed the ligamentum flavum and is therefore facing the epidural space and the wall of the dural sac: the smaller this distance, the lower the risk of accidental dural puncture. The not excessive protrusion of the needle within the epidural space depends on various factors, such as the subjective tactile perception of the operator and tissue parameters (peak force in the ligamentum flavum, drop force), and human factors, such as the position of the hand holding the needle, muscle cocontraction (which makes the wrist and finger joints of both hands rigid), and speed of needle insertion. Experts are able to control the protrusion of the needle in the epidural space by adjusting the pressure exerted on the needle–syringe–piston system, controlling the speed of the needle, and perceiving changes in force, while beginners do not have this ability [9].

These are the emblematic testimonies of young residents who had faced the epidural block in practice for the first time, after having followed a theoretical teaching module. Some examples are reported among those that significantly represented the most commonly expressed opinions.

> The main difficulty is finding the anatomical reference points blindly, so the difficulty in finding the inter-space when you don't feel it well but also sometimes when you do feel it: you think you are there and instead you are a bit shifted.

> The difficulties I encountered were: in directing the needle much more than in feeling the consistencies of the various tissues that the needle passes through. Several times it happened that the tutor pointed the needle and then I was the one to find the epidural space and I never found any difficulty.

> The difficulty probably lies in understanding when there is and when the increase in resistance begins more than then understanding when there is the loss of resistance, which is clearer. I found it also difficult to get a bit of experience in manual skills, so holding the needle well positioned, braking with the left hand, correctly advancing the needle. On the average the major difficulty is often in finding the intervertebral space and therefore finding the most correct space immediately.

> The main difficulty I encountered was related to the ability to recognize the tissues encountered during the advancement of the needle when the anatomical circumstances are not typical, for example when there is an unusual hardness of the ligamentum flavum that can be mistakenly exchanged for the bone!

> The difficulties I had were mainly the recognition of the various anatomical planes of the epidural technique and learning to control the needle with the non-dominant hand when I encountered a particularly dense ligamentum flavum.

After a month of practice in the delivery room, the main difficulties of the students have changed and seem more focused on the environment rather than the technique, although there are still some doubts about how to perform the technique in difficult cases:

> The main difficulty is performing the technique in patients who are in active labor and the pharmacological management in the conversion from analgesia during labor to anesthesia for cesarean section.

> As for the main difficulties I encountered, I mention the management of the pregnant patient with strong contractions especially, at an advanced stage of labor with significant dilation of the uterine cervix or with very frequent and very intense contractions with an increase in difficulty in performing the technique due to the low compliance from the parturient.

> In the early stages, the difficulty was the recognition of the anatomical structures and the interpretation of a normal back and progressively in the identification of the difficult back and the structures in the difficult back.

> I feel that I have developed a decent knowledge of drugs and indications, and the same goes for autonomy, although I cannot yet consider myself fully autonomous. With supervision, I am able to perform a simple block more or less safely. Technical difficulties obviously still remain in more complex spines, and in these cases, I have difficulty feeling autonomous. Not feeling autonomous yet is a specific difficulty encountered in patients where the ligamentum flavum is very hard or very soft, or those cases where you have to go in a lot with the needle to feel the difference between losses of resistance more than the clear loss of resistance and vice versa when you are already three or four centimeters in and there is a very hard ligamentum flavum, understanding the difference with the bone, fearing that pushing too much if it is not bone but ligamentum, you risk puncturing the dura mater.

In fact, during the training period, after getting the fundamentals of the technique, the main difficulties encountered by the novice are solving complex problems (such as in obese or scoliotic patients), learning and choosing the appropriate administration of analgesia, and how to deal with any complications. Among the complexities of this phase, the relationships with the patient, the environment, and the delivery room staff, which often may produce relational problems that are difficult to resolve for a novice, are certainly relevant.

## 4 General Principles

### 4.1 Premises

Teaching and learning in anesthesiology is a challenging and complex task because most of the teaching and learning takes place in a clinical setting, where patient safety and comfort must be balanced with the responsibility of training the resident. Teaching and learning epidural analgesia for labor can be particularly challenging because the patient may be experiencing severe pain and therefore may not be willing to be involved in the educational encounter. Moreover, the clinical context of a delivery room where relatives are present may not be a comfortable environment for teaching and learning. Epidural analgesia for labor can therefore be difficult to teach and learn in a clinical context and represents a challenge for both the teacher and the learner [10, 11].

Furthermore, it is important to keep in mind that the approach to medical skills has changed. Previously, the focus was mainly on teaching the clinical knowledge and procedural skills necessary to practice the specialist profession. Today, it is generally accepted that physicians must possess a broader body of knowledge, which includes not only clinical and procedural skills but also professional behaviors to ensure competence.

Medicine has indeed adapted another way of viewing skills, derived from aviation, dividing them into technical and nontechnical skills. Technical skills are those related to the role of a medical expert. Nontechnical skills (NTS) can be defined as "the cognitive, social, and personal resources that complement technical skills and contribute to the safe and efficient execution of tasks" [12]. The NTS for anesthesiologists, described in the anesthetists nontechnical skills (ANTS) document [13], include skills related to situation awareness, decision-making, communication, teamwork, leadership, and stress and emergency management.

For example, learning the technique of epidural analgesia in labor does not only mean learning to place an epidural catheter, but it is a complex task that involves theoretical, technical, behavioral, and relational knowledge.

## 4.2 Learning Skills

Anesthesia is a practical specialty, and few other educational situations offer the same opportunities for close mutual observation between a teacher and a learner regarding technical (in this case, the execution of the epidural) and behavioral (statements, opinions, interactions, and reactions under pressure) aspects. It is difficult for a teacher to hide their technical and managerial skills, and in the same way, the students cannot easily hide their knowledge, skills, and attitudes when confronted with a specific clinical situation, especially in the presence of a patient [14].

Although any anesthesia trainee enthusiastically desires to immediately practice the procedure, it would be good to remind them that the first fundamental and important step is to observe someone else performing it using their own consolidated skills. This "tutor observation" phase is the first of the stages that, according to Collins [15], a teacher should use to help their student to master a technical task. Collins' stages are as follows:

1. Demonstration Phase: during which the expert performs the task while the student observes.

2. Training Phase: the student is assisted by the expert who intervenes, where necessary, providing feedback.
3. Assistance Phase: the student tries to perform the task with the guidance of the expert, who gradually and intentionally increases the complexity of the work undertaken, while slowly decreasing the intervention.
4. Withdrawal Phase: the expert reduces their support, providing only occasional suggestions, refinements, or evaluations but allowing the student to proceed independently.

The tutorial functions have been well described by Wood et al. [16] and are:

Interest in the task: the tutor must try to motivate the student not only in the initial phase but also at any time of difficulty that the learner encounters.
Reducing degrees of freedom: the tutor tries to lighten the task based on the level of learning within the student's reach at that time.
Maintaining direction: the tutor encourages the student to maintain the path that leads him to the final goal and tries to keep his motivation high.
Highlighting crucial aspects: the tutor points out the critical aspects of the task to the student.
Controlling frustration: the tutor helps the student control the anxiety of achieving the goal.
Demonstration or modeling: the tutor proposes the solution by showing himself how it is done.

## 4.3 Learning Methods

The learning objectives of the epidural technique can be summarized as follows:

**Theoretical learning objectives**
- Understand the anatomy.
- Understand how a solution spreads in the epidural space.
- Know the risks and complications of epidural placement and how to manage them.
- Know the different local anesthetics and their use.
- Know the dosage of local anesthetics.
- Know the contraindications to epidural placement.

**Technical skill learning objectives**
- Know the materials.
- Use a correct aseptic technique.
- Use a safe method for epidural placement.
- Test the correct placement of the epidural.
- Use proper dressing.

**Nontechnical skill learning objectives**
- Leadership (assume leadership, guide the team).
- Communication (closed-loop, information).
- Teamwork (coordination, support).
- Task management (planning, preparing, setting priorities).
- Situation awareness (recognizing, understanding).
- Decision-making process (identifying options, reevaluating).

## 4.4 Theoretical Knowledge

In theory, practical learning should be preceded by classroom lessons and teaching sessions. The theoretical knowledge to be taught may vary depending on the institutes but generally includes at least one session on the anatomy of the epidural space and the theoretical principles of the technical methodology. These basic lessons can be integrated, within the training curriculum, with specific lessons concerning the pharmacological aspects and other aspects of obstetric anesthesia. It would be appropriate to provide learners with suitable teaching materials (books, handouts, videos, interactive online courses, etc.) and the opportunity to adequately discuss, in the classroom or with their tutor, unclear or more complex topics. This allows the tutor to verify the student's understanding of the theoretical foundations that will then be used in clinical practice.

## 4.5 Teaching and Learning Procedural Skills in the Clinical Setting

The literature has demonstrated the benefits of active experiential learning compared to traditional lectures, as "learning by doing" promotes an actual improvement in high-level thinking processes [17–19], greater retention of knowledge [18, 20], and a higher degree of student satisfaction [21].

In accordance with Dale's learning pyramid theory [22], learners remember 90% of what they have been told if they have been actively involved in a practical activity, i.e., if they have seen and done it. This is particularly applicable in the context of teaching medical procedures [23] and therefore also the epidural technique.

Teaching and learning practical procedural skills for the epidural technique in obstetrics, and especially for labor analgesia, represent a challenge in the clinical context as it involves learning the technique during labor. Therefore, it would be appropriate for basic technical skills to be practiced not directly on the patient, but with a simulator before starting training in the clinical setting.

There are several central neural block simulators, from the simple "greengrocer" model to high-fidelity devices (see Chapter "Epidural Simulators"). The important thing is that the trainee is able to practice procedural skills in a safe environment without the risk of harming the patient. It has been shown that simulation training for procedural skills improves knowledge and skills in both simple and more complex procedures [24]. Even on the simulator, it is possible to use the three-phase teaching technique, in which the educator first shows the procedure on the simulator without explaining it, while the learner observes. Subsequently, the educator repeats the procedure and at the same time systematically explains all the steps to the learner. Finally, the learner performs the procedure explaining all the steps to the educator. The last phase is repeated until the learner feels confident.

After theoretical preparation and simulator training, the learner can begin training in the clinical setting. The educator must supervise the learner, and the training must be guided by learning objectives. During the training, it is essential to provide feedback, which is the fundamental tool of effective clinical teaching. With feedback, the learner's strengths are reinforced, and errors can be corrected, while encouraging reflection and autonomous learning. It seems that feedback given at the end of the procedure is superior to that given during the procedure itself in improving short- and long-term memory of the practiced technique [25].

Providing feedback after performing the procedure also allows for discussion with the student away from potential judgments expressed by colleagues and patients or other healthcare professionals [26].

Learning and teaching effectiveness can be guided by learning curves and CUSUM evaluation (see Chapter "Learning Curves") which help the teacher to assess the competence of their student and decide when it is time to let them perform the procedure on their own.

## 4.6 Training in Nontechnical Skills

It is commonly believed that training in epidural technique concerns exclusively technical aspects and, subsequently, pharmacological aspects and how to deal with difficult cases or the treatment of possible complications. However, the success of the technique often also depends on the organizational and interdisciplinary communication skills of the anesthesiologist (nontechnical skills).

Examples of theoretical knowledge and technical skills are as follows: discussing which analgesic solution to use, summarizing the principles of treatment for local anesthetic toxicity, performing a neuraxial block, or recognizing an accidental intravenous administration in the epidural catheter.

Examples of nontechnical or behavioral skills are as follows: how to ask for informed consent for labor analgesia, how to discuss and plan a cesarean section with obstetric colleagues, how to manage the team in the case of postpartum hemorrhage, how to talk to the relatives, etc.

It is therefore essential, from the very beginning of practical training on the patient, that the teacher also takes care of the "relational aspects" of the epidural block.

For example, communication with the laboring woman and her family can be trained using simulated patients and simulating different scenarios with increasing difficulty, from information on the insertion of an epidural catheter to information on an adverse event.

It is certainly difficult to train for teamwork in relation to the insertion of an epidural catheter for labor analgesia in a clinical context. The laboring woman is suffering, the atmosphere can be tense, and training for teamwork along with technical skills in this situation may not be acceptable to the laboring woman. In this case, simulation can provide a safe learning environment where patients are not exposed or harmed and, moreover, offers the possibility of practicing repetitively.

Simulation-based training to develop and consolidate teamwork skills, using a variety of different scenarios, has already been widely proven to be effective for obstetric teams and should become part of the training for young anesthesiologists attending delivery rooms to learn the epidural technique and its clinical management [27–33].

Table 1 shows the nontechnical skills for anesthesiologists (ANTS) [34] and Table 2 its application to the epidural block.

## 4.7 Assessment of Learning

The assessment of learning (or competence) is an aspect that unfortunately does not receive enough attention in the teaching of the epidural block. Often, it is limited to counting how many epidurals the residents have performed or anecdotally noting that during the practical training period, the number of accidental dural punctures increases significantly, but considering this event as an inevitable price to pay. It has

**Table 1** Nontechnical skills in anesthesia (ANTS)

| |
|---|
| Task management |
| Planning and preparation |
| Prioritization |
| Provide and maintain standards |
| Identify and utilize resources |
| Teamwork |
| Coordinate activities with team members |
| Exchange of information |
| Use authority and assertiveness |
| Evaluate capabilities |
| Support others |
| Situation awareness |
| Gathering information |
| Recognize and understand |
| Anticipate |
| Decision-making |
| Identify options |
| Balance risks and select options |
| Reevaluate |

**Table 2** Nontechnical skills for epidural block execution

| ANTS | Example |
|---|---|
| *Task management* | |
| Planning and preparation | Interview with the patient before the block |
| Setting priorities | Decide what is best to do before, during, and immediately after the block (e.g., maternal, fetal monitoring) |
| Provide and maintain standards | Introduce yourself to the patient |
| Identify and utilize resources | Get help from a midwife or nurse in performing the block |
| *Teamwork* | |
| Coordinate activities with team members | Agree with staff on what and how to inform the patient during the procedure |
| Exchange of information | Obtain information on the progress of labor |
| Use authority and assertiveness | Exercise leadership during the execution of the block (the attention of the patient and healthcare professionals should be on the operator performing the block) |
| Evaluate capabilities | Own and collaborators' |
| Supporting others | Relating and communicating with relatives without excluding them |
| *Situation awareness* | |
| Gathering information | Knowing the patient's expectations |
| Recognizing and understanding | Recognizing when the patient is tired when the block execution times are excessively prolonged |
| Anticipating | Anticipating to the patient the sensations they will have during the block execution |
| *Making decisions* | |
| Identifying options | Knowing when it is time to discuss with the patient and colleagues alternatives in the case of technical difficulties |
| Balancing risks and selecting options | Knowing when to stop and interrupt the procedure when its execution is no longer tolerated by the patient |
| Reevaluating | Knowing how to repeat the procedure if in doubt and motivating the patient with the reasons |

been reported [35], but it is also a common experience and widespread opinion among teachers that not all residents receive adequate training before performing their first epidural in labor and that a formal assessment is rarely carried out at the end of their practical training to certify the skills acquired. Just as it is important to decide and describe which learning objectives to include in the training within the educational curriculum (knowledge, skills, and attitudes), it is equally important to decide how to evaluate them. The first question to consider is as follows: what is the purpose of our assessment? Is it a formative assessment aimed at promoting further learning or a summative assessment that aims to evaluate whether the trainee has the necessary competence to perform a specific medical activity without supervision?

Ideally, both types of assessment should be used: formative assessment during specialist training to guide learning and summative assessment at specific moments.

Assessment should be one of the fundamental stages of training [36] also because it contributes to shaping the ways in which trainees learn: if both technical execution and management and communication skills are assessed, the trainees will focus on both aspects and consider them both important factors for their professional life [37, 38].

Competence assessment should include not only the specialist role but also the roles of collaborator, communicator, manager, and professional. Ideally, the assessment of different roles should be included in a single assessment. The assessment should therefore include all three levels of competence: (1) knowledge and skills, (2) the ability to apply knowledge and skills, and (3) attitudes and personal abilities.

Assessment in a clinical environment is quite challenging, but it is important to ensure high-quality patient care. The assessment must reflect what trainees do in actual patient care. The issues related to learning assessment are extensively discussed in the Chapters "Assessing Learning" and "Learning Curves".

A particular assessment is that of a training program. Usually, Kirkpatrick's four-level evaluation model [39] is used for this purpose. The first level, or reaction level, measures the satisfaction of participants/learners with the training/intervention. The second level, the learning level, describes the degree of change in the learner's knowledge, skills, and attitudes. The third level is the behavioral or organizational level, which illustrates the impact on clinical practice: do programs follow guidelines? Are there changes in routine within the organization? Finally, the fourth level represents the outcome level for patients. It describes the benefits for patients, such as a lower incidence of dural punctures. Evaluating a program at all four levels is challenging and requires resources.

## 5 The Educator and the Learning Environment

Teaching epidural analgesia in labor is challenging, and the educator must be more than a medical expert to be successful. However, many physicians in teaching hospitals have not received formal training on how to teach and base their teaching on their own past learning experiences [40].

To achieve successful teaching, institutions should provide support and training to their clinical teachers. The skills that make an excellent clinical teacher are outlined in Table 3 [41].

Table 4 shows a simple scheme for daily teaching described by Neher [42] that highlights how to give feedback and facilitate learning. The clinical teacher must be a content expert and able to create a positive learning environment but must also have good listening skills and enthusiasm for teaching.

In a large review of studies published from 1909 to 2006 on the characteristics of good teachers in the medical field [41], as many as 480 descriptors of the characteristics of a good clinical teacher were identified. The most frequently cited characteristics in the literature are as follows:

(a) Characteristics of the physician as a teacher.

**Table 3** Competencies that make an excellent clinical teacher

| |
|---|
| Passion for teaching |
| Clear, organized, approachable, supportive, and compassionate |
| Ability to establish rapport, provide guidance and feedback, demonstrate integrity, and respect for others |
| Demonstrating clinical competence |
| Utilizes planning and orientation strategies |
| Possesses a wide repertoire of teaching methods |
| Engages in self-assessment and reflection |
| Draws on multiple forms of knowledge, addressing teaching to the level of knowledge of learners |

**Table 4** The five important steps to facilitate learning

| |
|---|
| Phase 1 Create a safe learning environment. Let the trainee manage and guide the procedure |
| Phase 2 Encourage the trainee to explain and speak aloud during the procedure. Gently encourage or correct during the procedure |
| Phase 3 Guide the trainee to learn and understand general rules |
| Phase 4 Reinforce what has been done well |
| Phase 5 Correct the errors. Encourage self-assessment |

- Demonstrates knowledge, competence, and mastery of the subject.
- Demonstrates clinical competence, clinical acumen, clinical reasoning ability, correlation and synthesis skills, diagnostic competence, and technical competence.
- Demonstrates enthusiasm for medicine and their specialization.

(b) Characteristics of the teacher.
- Maintains a positive learning climate, respecting and supporting students.
- Creates a facilitating and comfortable learning environment.
- Respects trainees, considering them as colleagues.
- Has a genuine interest in students and cares for them and is ready to listen to their problems, aware of their needs and issues, and curious about their experiences.
- Provides a safe environment and corrects mistakes without belittling the person.

(c) Human characteristics.
- Is a good communicator and promotes open communication.
- Has good interpersonal communication skills.
- Has good listening skills.
- Has the ability to express oneself clearly and persuasively.

**Acknowledgments** We thank the following colleagues for the information regarding the state of the art of teaching epidural technique in their centers and their countries.

Peter Kranke, University of Würzburg, Germany.

Roshan Fernando, University College London Hospitals NHS Foundation Trust, London, UK.

Emilia Guash, Hospital Universitario La Paz, Madrid, Spain.
Bendan Carvalho, Stanford University Medical Center, USA.
Thierry Girard, University of Basel, Switzerland.
Elena Bignami, Azienda Ospedaliero-Universitaria di Parma, Italy.

## References


1. Bromage PR. Teaching techniques. In: Bromage PR, editor. Epidural analgesia. Philadelphia: WB Saunders; 1978. p. 716–7.
2. Chuan A, Jeyaratnam B, Fathil S, Ferraro LH, Kessow A, Lim YC, et al. Education in regional anesthesia collaboration (ERAC) group. Non-fellowship regional anesthesia training and assessment: an international Delphi study on a consensus curriculum. Reg Anesth Pain Med. 2021;46(10):867–73. https://doi.org/10.1136/rapm-2021-102934.
3. Training Requirements for the Specialty of Anaesthesiology, European Standards of Postgraduate Medical Specialist Training, European Union of Medical Specialists, 2022.
4. Grantcharov TP, Reznick RK. Teaching procedural skills. BMJ. 2008;336:1129–31. https://doi.org/10.1136/bmj.39517.686956.47.
5. Smith TS, Johannsson HE, Sadler C. Trials of labour: can simulation make a difference to obstetric anaesthetic training? Curr Anaesth Crit Care. 2005;16:289–96. https://doi.org/10.1016/j.cacc.2005.11.011.
6. Aggarwal R, Darzi A. Technical-skills training in the 21st century. N Engl J Med. 2006;355:2695–6. https://doi.org/10.1056/NEJMe068179.
7. Watterson LM, Hyde S, Bajenov S, Kennedy SE. The training environment of junior anaesthetic registrars learning epidural labour analgesia in Australian Teaching Hospitals. Anaesth Intensive Care. 2007;35:38–46. https://doi.org/10.1177/0310057X0703500133.
8. Isaacs R, Wee MYK, Dubey VN, Vaughan N. A survey of trainees' perspectives on epidural training in the United Kingdom. Glob Anaesth Perioper Med. 2015;4:121–4. https://doi.org/10.15761/GAPM.1000130.
9. Senac T, Lelevé A, Moreau R, Krähenbühl L, Sigwalt F, Bauer C. Skill assessment of an epidural anesthesia using the PeriSIM simulator. In: IEEE transactions on medical robotics and bionics, vol. 3. Piscataway, NJ: IEEE; 2021. p. 106–14.
10. Spencer J. Learning and teaching in the clinical environment. BMJ. 2003;326:591–4. https://doi.org/10.1136/bmj.326.7389.591.
11. Ramani S, Leinster S. AMEE Guide no. 34: teaching in the clinical environment. Med Teach. 2008;30(4):347–64. https://doi.org/10.1080/01421590802061613.
12. Flin RH, O'Connor P, Crichton M. Safety at the sharp end: a guide to non-technical skills. Ashgate, England: Aldershot; 2008.
13. Fletcher GCL, McGeorge P, Flin RH, Glavin RJ, Maran NJ. The role of non-technical skills in anaesthesia: a review of current literature. Br J Anaesth. 2022;88:418–29. https://doi.org/10.1093/bja/88.3.418.
14. Cantillon P, Wood P. ABC of learning and teaching in medicine. London: BMJ Books; 2010.
15. Collins A, Brown JS, Holum A. Cognitive apprenticeship: making thinking visible. Am Educ. 1991;15:6–11.
16. Wood D, Bruner JS, Ross G. The role of tutoring in problem solving. J Child Psychol Psychiatry. 1976;17:89–100. https://doi.org/10.1111/j.1469-7610.1976.tb00381.x.
17. Kulik JA, Kulik CLC. College teaching. In: Peterson PL, Walberg HJ, editors. Research on teaching: concepts, findings, and implications. Berkeley: McCutcheon; 1979.
18. Smith DG. College classroom interactions and critical thinking. J Educ Psychol. 1977;69:180–90. https://doi.org/10.1037/0022-0663.69.2.180.
19. McKinney K, Graham-Buxton M. The use of collaborative learning groups in the large class: is it possible? Teach Sociol. 1993;21:403–8.

20. Rau W, Heyl BS. Humanizing the college classroom: collaborative learning and social organization among students. Teach Sociol. 1990;18:141–55.
21. Bligh DA. What's the use of lectures? Harmondsworth: Penguin Books; 1972.
22. Wagner RW. Edgar Dale: professional. Theory Pract. 1970;9:89–95.
23. Bosse HM, Mohr J, Buss B, Krautter M, Weyrich P, Herzog W, et al. The benefit of repetitive skills training and frequency of expert feedback in the early acquisition of procedural skills. BMC Med Educ. 2015;15:22. https://doi.org/10.1186/s12909-015-0286-5.
24. Lorello GR, Cook DA, Johnson RL, Brydges R. Simulation-based training in anaesthesiology: a systematic review and meta-analysis. BJA. 2014;112:231–45. https://doi.org/10.1093/bja/aet414.
25. Lean LL, Hong RYS, Ti LK. End-task versus in-task feedback to increase procedural learning retention during spinal anaesthesia training of novices. Adv Health Sci Educ Theory Pract. 2017;22:713–21. https://doi.org/10.1007/s10459-016-9703-8.
26. Garwood J, Wilkinson B. Teaching trainees neuraxial anaesthesia. What is the evidence? J Anaesth Intensive Care Med. 2020;10:555791. https://doi.org/10.19080/JAICM.2020.10.555791.
27. Draycott T, Sibanda T, Owen L, Akande V, Winter C, Reading S, et al. Does training in obstetric emergencies improve neonatal outcome? BJOG. 2006;113:177–82. https://doi.org/10.1111/j.1471-0528.2006.00800.x.
28. Kariya N, Kawasaki Y, Okutani H, Kaneko T, Ueki R, Hirose M. Effects of simulation study of high neuraxial block during epidural analgesia for labor pain on pre/posttest evaluation in junior clinical trainees. Anaesth Pain Med. 2020;10:e100045. https://doi.org/10.5812/aapm.100045.
29. Robertson B, Schumacher L, Gosman G, Kanfer R, Kelley M, DeVita M. Simulation-based crisis team training for multidisciplinary obstetric providers. Simul Healthc. 2009;4:77–83. https://doi.org/10.1097/SIH.0b013e31819171cd.
30. Freeth D, Ayida G, Berridge EJ, Mackintosh N, Norris B, Sadler C, et al. Multidisciplinary obstetric simulated emergency scenarios (MOSES): promoting patient safety in obstetrics with teamwork-focused interprofessional simulations. J Contin Educ Health Prof. 2009;29:98–104. https://doi.org/10.1002/chp.20018.
31. Draycott T, Crofts J. Structured team training in obstetrics and its impact on outcome. Fetal Matern Med Rev. 2006;17:229–37. https://doi.org/10.1017/S0965539506001793.
32. Crofts JF, Ellis D, Draycott TJ, Winter C, Hunt LP, Akande VA. Change in knowledge of midwives and obstetricians following obstetric emergency training: a randomised controlled trial of local hospital, simulation Centre and teamwork training. BJOG. 2007;114:1534–41. https://doi.org/10.1111/j.1471-0528.2007.01493.x.
33. Gum L, Greenhill J, Dix K. Clinical simulation in maternity (CSiM): Interprofessional learning through simulation team training. Qual Saf Health Care. 2010;19:e19. https://doi.org/10.1136/qshc.2008.030767.
34. Yee B, Naik VN, Joo HS, Savoldelli GL, Chung DY, Houston PL, et al. Nontechnical skills in anesthesia crisis management with repeated exposure to simulation-based education. Anesthesiology. 2005;103:241–8. https://doi.org/10.1097/00000542-200508000-00006.
35. Watterson LM, Hyde S, Bajenov S, Kennedy SE. The training environment of junior anaesthetic registrars learning epidural labour analgesia in Australian Teaching Hospitals. Anaesth Intensive Care. 2007;35:38–45. https://doi.org/10.1177/0310057X0703500133.
36. Ten Cate O. Entrustability of professional activities and competency-based training. Med Educ. 2005;39:1176–7. https://doi.org/10.1111/j.1365-2929.2005.02341.x.
37. Norcini J, Burch V. Workplace-based assessment as an educational tool: AMEE Guide no 31. Med Teach. 2007;29:855–71. https://doi.org/10.1080/01421590701775453.
38. Grant J. Learning needs assessments: assessing the need. BMJ. 2002;324:156–9. https://doi.org/10.1136/bmj.324.7330.156.
39. Kirkpatrick DL. Evaluating training programs. San Francisco: Beret-Koehler; 1998.

40. Van der Hem-Stokroos NH, Daelmans HF, Van der Vleuten CP, Haarman HJ, Scherphier AL. The impact of multi-faceted educational structuring on learning effectiveness in a surgical clerkship. Med Educ. 2004;38:879–86. https://doi.org/10.1111/j.1365-2929.2004.01899.x.
41. Surkin G, Wagner E, Harris I, Shiffer R. What makes a good clinical teacher in medicine? A review of the literature. Acad Med. 2008;83:452–66. https://doi.org/10.1097/ACM.0b013e31816bee61.
42. Neher JO, Gordon KC, Meyer B, Stevens N. A five-step "Microskills" model of clinical teaching. J Am Board Fam Pract. 1992;5:419–24.

# Epidural Simulators

Emanuele Capogna

Every teacher, during their career, has certainly sought the best way to have their students experience the sensation of loss of resistance, using materials already present in the operating room or easily available and at a low cost.

For example, any piece of polystyrene (Styrofoam) or other lightweight and porous plastic material (polyethylene), commonly used for packaging, can be used to demonstrate and have the student experience the sensation of "a loss of resistance" when inserting the epidural needle-syringe complex inside one of these materials. Some offer resistance to the needle's progression sufficiently comparable to that of the ligamentum flavum and are therefore suitable for describing the difference between an "increase" and a "loss" of resistance.

Unfortunately, for most of these "rudimentary simulators," we have no trace except anecdotal, nor do we have any idea how effectively they actually work and how much they can be suggested as standard teaching models.

## 1 The "Greengrocer" Model

"Place a clean potato of adequate size in a cup, so that it is firmly wedged by the edge. The cup must be placed on a solid surface and the Tuohy needle must be advanced as usual. The resistance to the advancement of the Tuohy needle through the potato is similar to that of the ligamentum flavum and the loss of resistance when the needle emerges through the opposite side of the potato is very similar to that experienced when entering the epidural space. The saline solution descends into the cup" (Fig. 1). This was published by Tuckey in the late 1990s [1] and

E. Capogna (✉)
European School of Obstetric Anesthesia, Maternal and Neonatal Simulation Center EESOA, Rome, Italy
e-mail: ema.capogna@gmail.com

© The Author(s), under exclusive license to Springer Nature Switzerland AG 2024

G. Capogna (ed.), *How to Teach the Epidural Block in Obstetric Anesthesia*, https://doi.org/10.1007/978-3-031-70211-2_2

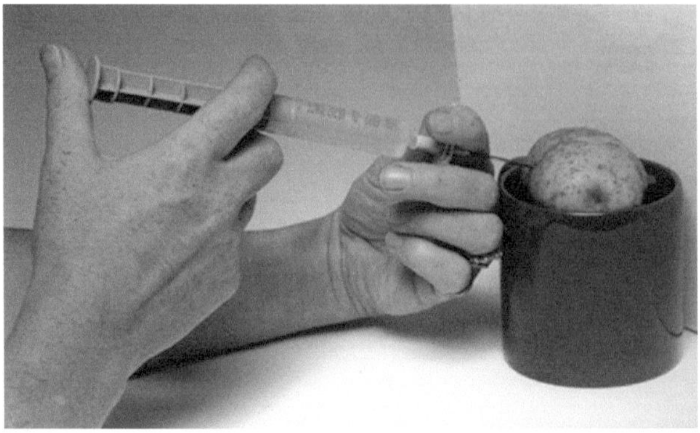

**Fig. 1** A potato is placed in a cup and the Tuohy needle advanced. The resistance to the advance of the Tuohy needle through the potato feels similar to the resistance of the ligamentum flavum and the loss of resistance as the needle emerges through the opposite side of the potato feels very similar to that experienced on entering the epidural space. The saline drops into the cup. (From [1] with permission)

approved by the great master Philip Bromage in a subsequent letter to the article, in which he also gave his recipe, starting from the potato, for a homemade spinal block simulator [2].

Ten years earlier, Leighton [3] had proposed the "greengrocer" model, probably one of the simplest and most economical epidural simulator models ever developed.

It consists of a slice of sandwich bread, a banana, and a balloon embedded in a polyurethane foam surgical headrest and covered by a transparent adhesive plastic bag. These layers simulate the skin, subcutaneous tissue, and ligamentum flavum.

According to the authors, the banana can be reused on average about 30 times. A hidden balloon represents the dura mater, and its rupture is used to indicate an accidental dural puncture. This model is very simple, easily reproducible, and low cost, but it does not recreate a very accurate sensation of human tissue. If sufficient pressure is not exerted on the piston of the epidural needle, its bevel tends to be obstructed by the banana pulp, and therefore, the sensation of loss of resistance is never experienced. Moreover, air must be used; otherwise, the bread becomes soaked with water. But the biggest limitation of this model is that the "bone" is not represented, making it possible for the needle to penetrate and advance, unrealistically, from any angle or position. Another model described in the literature is one consisting of a lemon at one end of which is attached a glass bottle or a surgical glove filled with water (in this case, an accidental dural puncture is also to be simulated) [4] (Fig. 2). In this simple model, the "skin puncture" is reproduced by the lemon peel near the needle insertion, the "resistances of the supraspinous and interspinous ligaments" by the lemon pulp, and the resistance of the "ligamentum flavum" by the thickness of the distal wall of the lemon peel, and finally, the "loss of resistance in the epidural space" is represented by the further progression and stopping of the needle that passes through the distal portion of the lemon peel but stops before puncturing the water-filled glove.

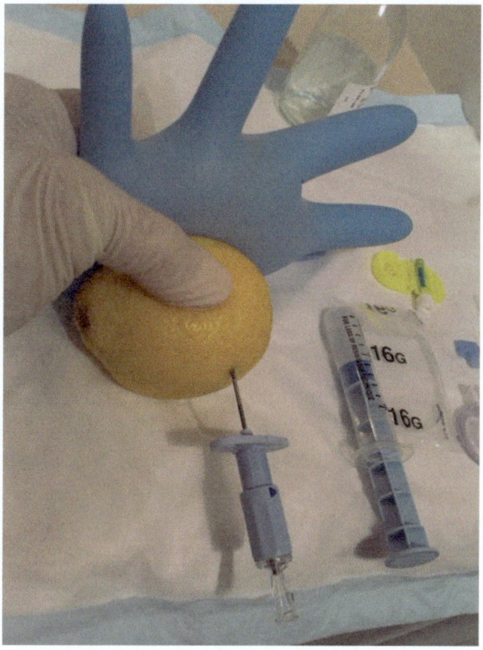


**Fig. 2** Lemon with opposed surgical glove distended with water to demonstrate "cerebrospinal fluid backflow" when penetrated by "needle through needle" spinal needle. (From [4] with permission)

Other fruits (orange, green melon, and kiwi) have also been used for this type of teaching, but it seems, according to the experts who have tried them, that the banana is the most appropriate [5].

## 2 Anthropomorphic-Based Simulators

Epidural "mannequin-type" simulators are three-dimensional anthropomorphic models that reproduce the anatomical structures that the anesthesiologist traverses with the needle during the execution of the epidural anesthesia technique, so that the learner can learn from the tactile experience on the simulator what the right pressure to apply is to perform the maneuver and how to locate the epidural space.

This simulator type is based on plastic material models, which are not computerized and generally do not contain mechanical or electronic parts.

They are portable, easy to set up and use, and some even have physically palpable anatomical landmarks.

They generally contain solid structures inside to represent the lumbar vertebrae, and their surface, which reproduces the morphology of the patient's lumbar area, is covered by an artificial synthetic skin. Inside the simulator, there is often a "dural sac" made of rubber or silicone, fillable with a liquid to simulate the cerebrospinal fluid. Some of these simulators can be used in different positions, to recreate the sitting or lateral decubitus position.

Examples available on the market are the M43 3B simulator from Kyoto Kagaku (Fig. 3), the lumbar epidural injection simulator from Pharmabotics Ltd., the adult lumbar epidural injection and lumbar puncture simulator from Shengyuan Medical Devices, the Life/form® spinal injection simulator from Nasco (Fig. 4), the epidural simulator from Erler Zimmer R100777 (Fig. 5), and the P61 epidural and spinal injection device from 3B Scientific (Fig. 6).

One of the main limitations of this simulator type is that they do not always faithfully reproduce the anatomical characteristics of all the layers that the needle must pass through (skin, subcutaneous fat, supraspinous and interspinous ligaments, and ligamentum flavum), and sometimes, the solid plastic structure used to represent the vertebrae does not accurately reproduce the vertebral arch and other possible bony parts that may be encountered during needle insertion.

These simulators are evaluated or validated by groups of so-called experts (often anesthesiologists with experience of a few hundred blocks) who provide a personal judgment on the quality and realism of the sensations perceived as the epidural needle passes through the various layers of the simulator. The average user evaluation of commercially available simulators, based on subjective scales, has been reported as widely variable, usually reaching average or low scores. Although these simulators can reproduce the sensation of loss of resistance quite well, they often fail to reproduce the sensation of increased resistance due to the ligamentum flavum, false losses of resistance in the tissues in front of the ligamentum flavum, and bone contact, especially in those simulators where the bone is represented by an amorphous plastic compound [6, 7].

The limitations of this type of evaluation with subjective scales are evidenced by a blind study [8] that compared the realism of different epidural simulators. One of the evaluations concerned how plausible the lumbar landmark points were to palpation, and the study reported that some participants believed that palpating the reference points offered by the simulator containing a banana was the most realistic, despite, obviously, there being no structures similar to vertebrae to palpate!

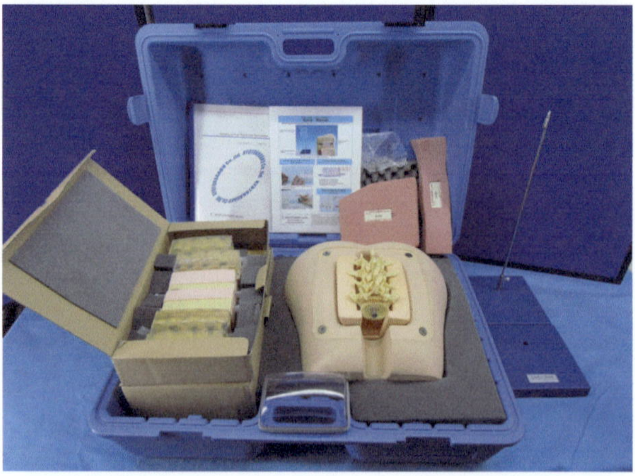

**Fig. 3** The simulator M43 3B (Kyoto Kagaku)

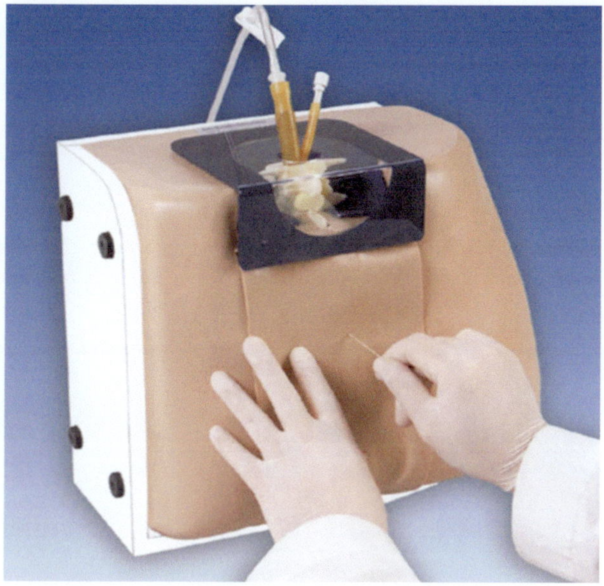

**Fig. 4** The Life/form simulator (Nasco)

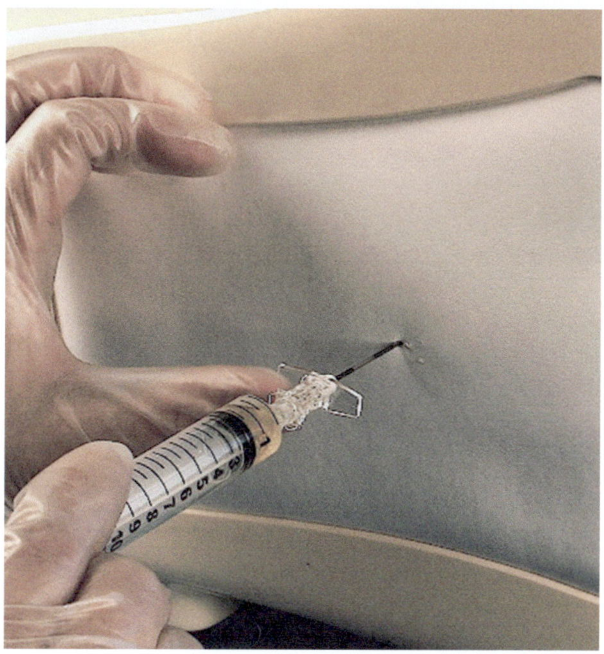

**Fig. 5** The simulator Erler Zimmer R100777

In an attempt to more faithfully reproduce the tissues traversed by the needle, various custom-made, reusable prototypes have been proposed [9], but their validation in clinical practice has never been reported.

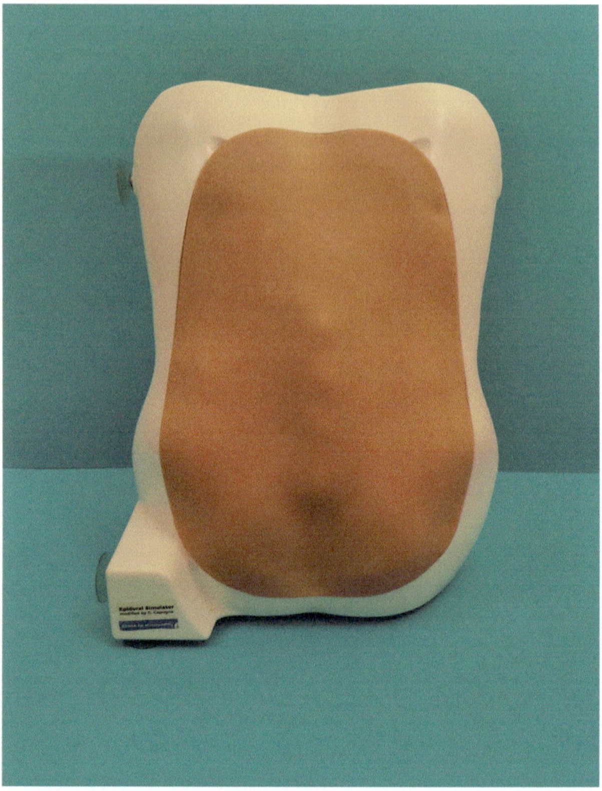

**Fig. 6** The simulator P61 (3B Scientific)

Another alternative to expensive and not always adequately realistic commercial epidural simulators is to build a homemade epidural simulator, using low-cost materials such as a "memory foam" pillow, a plastic skeleton model, and other easily available materials [10].

Unfortunately, even these "homemade" models have never been validated nor has their educational use been reported except in the introductory published study.

Another way that has been proposed to make the "simulator tissues" more realistic is to use a 3D printer. Some authors have built an epidural simulator using Free/Libre/open-source software (FLOS) [11]. Unfortunately, currently, these printed models lack realism in superficial palpation due to the softness of the gelatin solution used. Moreover, the use of perishable materials such as gelatin and psyllium requires continuous replacement both for material deterioration and because the signs of needle tracks persist in the models after use.

## 2.1 The Modified P61 Simulator: The Epidural Module$^{EESOA}$

To overcome the limitations of commercial simulators, our study group has created and validated an epidural simulator by modifying the internal structure of one available on the market (epidural simulator P61 from 3B Scientific) (Fig. 6), with neoprene and silicone-based materials.

The simulator module we propose is a semi-handcrafted reproducible artifact that effectively mimics patients' lumbar epidural region, which, unpredictably for both the operator and their tutor, can have different consistencies in their ligamentous or subcutaneous systems, with varying thicknesses and distances from the skin. Furthermore, the material used, after repeated attempts, becomes impregnated with the saline solution used for the epidural technique and effectively simulates the tissue imbibition that occurs in living beings when repeated attempts of injection are made. The material also effectively simulates false loss of resistance that can be encountered if the needle is stopped before the ligamentum flavum, and the presence of the bone model realistically reproduces bone contact in all its variations.

One of the problems with commercial mannequin simulators is that they are generally designed based on expert opinions but not on actual recorded data. In contrast, in our case, we were able to validate the modifications we made inside the P61 epidural simulator by measuring and comparing the pressure curves and forces exerted by the operator on the mannequin to those obtained on living beings in previous studies.

The insertion of our Module$^{EESOA}$ within the chassis of the 3B Scientific P61 epidural simulator has proven to be able to realistically reproduce the anatomical characteristics of the layers that the needle must pass through to reach the epidural space, as demonstrated by the similarity between the simulator's pressure curves and those of humans and the pressure values recorded during needle insertion [12].

The modified P61 simulators, with the insertion of the Module$^{EESOA}$, are routinely used in our simulation center and at some Italian specialization schools [13].

Daily teaching practice has shown that the insertion of the Epidural Module$^{EESOA}$ in the P61 simulator model from 3B Scientific improves its realism and educational performance, leaving all its original functions unchanged: possibility of performing lumbar, spinal, or CSE epidural technique in both sitting and lateral positions, with median or paramedian approach, accidental dural puncture.

In the Appendix, the method and materials needed to create an Epidural Module$^{EESOA}$ are described.

### 2.2 Anthropomorphic Model-Based Simulators Ultrasound Compatible

These simulators allow ultrasound scanning, making it possible to visualize internal structures before puncture and estimate the depth and position of the epidural space (Fig. 7).

Examples of these simulators are the Simulab Corporation's mannequin trainer for puncture/epidural, compatible with ultrasound and containing palpable lumbar vertebrae with spinous processes and iliac crests, the Blue Phantom distributed by 3B Scientific for lumbar and epidural puncture that can be used with any standard probe and supports sitting or lateral decubitus, and the Adam,Rouilly mannequin for

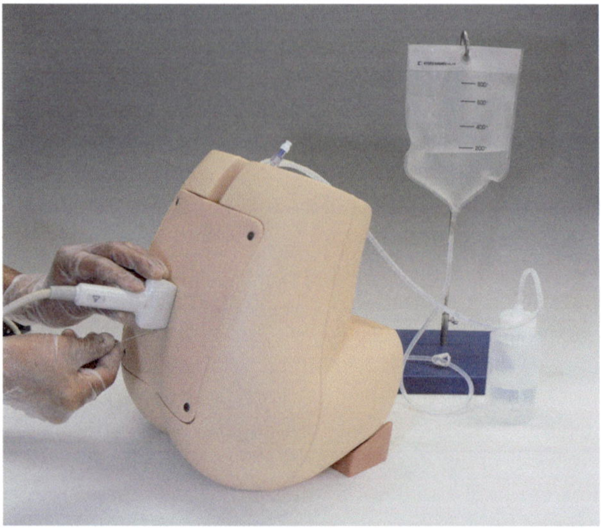

**Fig. 7** Ultrasound compatible epidural simulator

regional anesthesia simulation, which is a complete mannequin representing the upper body and supports epidural insertion at all vertebral levels.

Like standard simulators, echogenic ones are also expensive, so low-cost prototypes have been proposed as an alternative. For example, a 3D model reconstructed from a cadaveric computed tomography scan and then recreated using Mimics software and 3D printed with nylon plastic has been hypothesized. This prototype was evaluated by a team of trainees who reported "positive feedback" [14].

## 3 Haptic Simulators

The first mechanical simulator was created in 1990 by Daykin and Bacon and called the Portex epidural injection simulator [15]. It worked by inserting a Tuohy needle through a spring-loaded device that produced frictional resistance forces similar to those of tissues on a needle. At a certain depth, corresponding to the average distance between the skin and the epidural space, the needle opened a solenoid valve that interrupted the resistance. It was a relatively simple device, without computerized control. The instrument was validated by a subsequent study that compared the pressure curves recorded in vivo in obstetric patients with those of the in vitro simulator [16].

Currently, the alternative to "mannequin-type" simulators is represented by haptic simulators, usually associated with 3D computerized images that combine a physical interface with a virtual reality visualization of the needle's advancement.

As is known, people can quickly and accurately identify an object through touch, and haptic perception is the process of recognizing objects through proprioception and touch. It is derived from the combination of tactile perception of the object on the surface of the fingertips, interpreting its shape and nature in relation to proprioception (perception of one's body position relative to the object itself).

This recognition occurs through an exploration procedure, for example, by moving the fingers on the object's surface or holding it entirely in hand. Haptic perception is also derived from the forces experienced during object palpation.

In haptic perception, therefore, there is a conscious processing of the simple elements perceived, adding them together to obtain a structural whole.

Haptic interfaces are therefore devices or robotic systems that provide the user with tactile kinesthetic sensations (tactile feedback) or force (force feedback) and serve to guide the user on the position and nature of objects in virtual space.

In this simulator type, haptic forces are derived from data obtained during the insertion of an epidural needle from the skin to the epidural space on human or animal cadavers, or suggested by expert opinions. A 3D video can display the needle's position overlaid on previously recorded real magnetic resonance images [17].

Most of the haptic simulators reported in the literature are unfortunately not commercially available, often being prototypes; some are patented but, in general, have never been used in the current practice of clinical teaching [18–20].

The Mediseus from 3D Systems, one of the few commercially available, uses a haptic interface that provides forces and stiffness simulating the real interaction between the needle and the tissue and a virtual environment that allows real-time visualization of the needle insertion on the computer monitor. This simulator has unfortunately been criticized for its lack of realism [21].

More recently, prototypes have been described that integrate a haptic sensor with virtual reality [22, 23] (Fig. 8).

Among these is a simulator that also provides a method for training and evaluating residents through virtual reality [24]. A virtual tutor, after explaining and

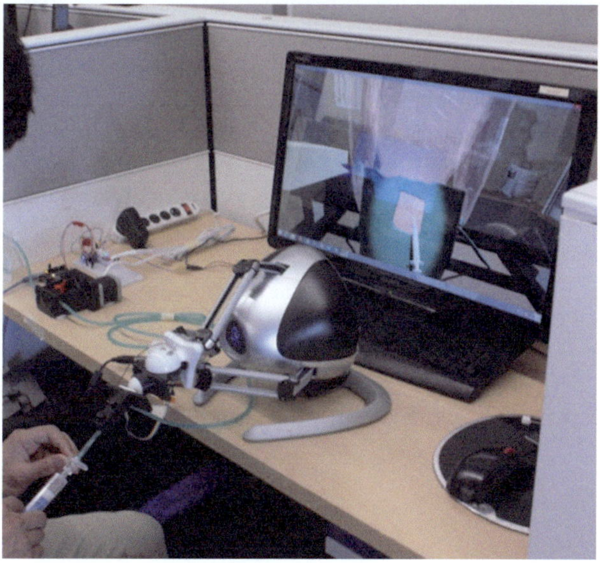

**Fig. 8** Integrated virtual reality and haptic simulator

performing the epidural block, invites the student to perform the block in successive steps, controlled by the tutor himself. The student performs the block through a haptic device connected to the epidural needle and syringe. The virtual tutor guides the resident through each phase of the block, one at a time, until the completion of the epidural or its failure. At the end of the process, an evaluation card is displayed. It can also be used in the variant that involves identifying the epidural space with ultrasound.

The use of haptic simulators has also been proposed as a complement to the training programs of doctors in training. For example, the PeriSIM haptic simulator [25] has been proposed and presented as a tool for evaluating the technical skills of anesthesia residents with a "machine learning" approach, identifying a series of quantifiable variables that allow categorizing the operator as an expert or novice. For example, some of the measurable variables from this simulator are as follows: the 3D position of the needle bevel, the forces applied to the needle tip, the insertion angle, the number of insertions, the number of bone contacts, the position of the bevel at the end of the procedure, the force exerted on the plunger, the average speed of needle introduction, its acceleration, the needle overshooting, etc.

## 4 Comparative Considerations

The mannequin simulators currently on the market are easy to install, portable, and usually cheaper. The main advantage is that mannequins are physical and not virtual, making them more similar to the reality of the patient.

For example, mannequins often contain a spinal canal filled with saline solution that can leak in the case of dura perforation, and this not only makes the event more realistic but also allows the operator to remove the skin and look inside the simulator.

One disadvantage of mannequin simulators is that the accuracy of needle insertion forces through artificial rubber or plastic skin is difficult to measure. Most insertion forces have been designed based on the opinions of doctors who have tried an insertion and provided feedback, but they are not based on actual recorded data.

Moreover, it is difficult for mannequins to contain all the correct anatomical layers, such as skin, subcutaneous fat, various ligaments, dura mater, the epidural space, as well as an accurate reproduction of the vertebral lamina and bony processes.

Generally, they also cannot adapt to patient variations, such as obesity, pregnancy, and age, all factors that can influence the operator's tactile appreciation.

Computerized simulators have two main advantages: haptic technology and real-time 3D visualizations.

The goal of haptic devices is to recreate forces to simulate ligaments, tissues, and bones, and this technology has certainly improved significantly in recent years.

The advantage of 3D virtual reality is that it allows you to see the needle from all angles and clearly visualize its position relative to the internal spinal anatomy.

While this feature can be highly educational, it is also equally unrealistic, and its use does not allow for training in blind insertion and progression of the needle, as will occur in the real patient.

The haptic simulator allows for the insertion of an unlimited number of needles without leaving marks from previous attempts, and the sensation is not compromised by the effect of multiple attempts on the physical structure of the mannequin. It also allows for various approaches to the epidural space, including midline and paramedian approaches at multiple spinal levels.

Computerized models can record and reproduce epidural attempts and provide automatic feedback on the results obtained and a score. However, they are more expensive than a mannequin and difficult to find commercially.

## 5 Educational Effectiveness of Epidural Simulators

The key elements of simulation-based training, such as repeated practice, goal feedback, and debriefing, combined with the fact that patients are not exposed to the intervention of absolute beginners, make simulation the ideal model for preliminary teaching of regional anesthesia and therefore also of the epidural technique.

American guidelines for anesthesia residency accreditation have set a time frame for simulation to be dedicated each year, and simulation is one of the elements required for maintaining board certification [26]. In Italy, simulation is also among the elements of national training courses and pathways of SIAARTI.

A large meta-analysis providing a detailed quantitative and critical narrative analysis of the evidence generated over the last 40 years [27] has demonstrated strong scientific evidence for the value of simulation-based training, although, due to the insufficient methodological approach of some studies, the direct benefits to the patient are lower than expected [28].

The methodological insufficiency of studies concerning simulation is also lamented by another meta-analysis (which, however, refers to regional anesthesia and not specifically to epidural simulation) stating that the scientific evidence in this field is unfortunately still preliminary and limited [29].

The problem is that, usually, participants in these types of studies, when assigned to the group using simulation, receive more hours of training than participants serving as controls. On the other hand, even if we know that adding simulation training automatically entails additional training, we cannot assume that this automatically leads to the acquisition of new knowledge or skills. In practice, studies comparing simulation to a standardized and consolidated method would be desirable.

And this is also why we can read controversial results among various studies. For example, one study reported that using a simple epidural simulator model like the "fruit vendor" type can be just as effective as a highly technological and very expensive commercial model that combines a physical interface with a virtual reality visualization of needle progression [30]. Another study found no differences in the acquisition of technical skills in performing epidural block between anesthesia residents who had undergone training with a low-fidelity simulator (banana) compared to those who had practiced with mental imagery technique [31].

Other studies, however, have demonstrated the effectiveness of using the simulator as a teaching tool [32, 33].

It is interesting to note that in a survey of anesthesia residents in the United Kingdom, more than 80% of respondents would recommend the educational use of such a tool, even though only 53% had used it prior to the interview [34].

# 6 Appendix. the Epidural Module[EESOA]

## 6.1 Required Materials

A complete P61 simulator from 3B Scientific, commercially available.

A tube of transparent anti-mold silicone sealant, such as Sil-Universale D2391 from Bostick, in a 280 mL package, available at hardware stores.

A black closed-cell neoprene tube for covering and insulating hydraulic pipes, used for outdoor purposes, available at hardware stores or plumbing shops.

## 6.2 Module Construction

After 3D scanning a lumbar spine model (Sawbones model SKU#1323–3), we adapted it in a one-piece box of adequate size to be inserted into the epidural simulator.

A groove for housing an endoscope was also created within the module to allow the trainee to observe the path of the needle and catheter within the epidural space. A printable file was then created in .stl format that allows the model to be 3D printed, using sls technology, by using nylon pa12 (the file is available at www.eesoa.com/episimu).

After having printed the module, shape the silicone from the lower edge and the anteroinferior surface of the cranial vertebra to the upper edge and the posterosuperior surface of the caudal vertebra, making sure that the thickness is greater in the center of the interlaminar foramen and smaller at the edges and that it also covers the bony laminae of the vertebral arch for a few millimeters (Fig. 9).

This silicone layer represents the ligamentum flavum, as silicone provides a tactile sensation similar to that of the ligamentum flavum, providing a hard-elastic consistency for needle insertion and giving the typical tactile sensation when penetrated.

Allow the silicone to dry for 12–24 h.

Using a kitchen blender, reduce the neoprene tube into pieces about 1.5–2 cm in size and mix them in a plastic bowl with the transparent silicone sealant in a 3:1 ratio to obtain a dense and homogeneous mixture that can be penetrated by the needle with little or no resistance: this layer represents the interspinous ligament, the paravertebral muscle fascia, and the multifidus muscle.

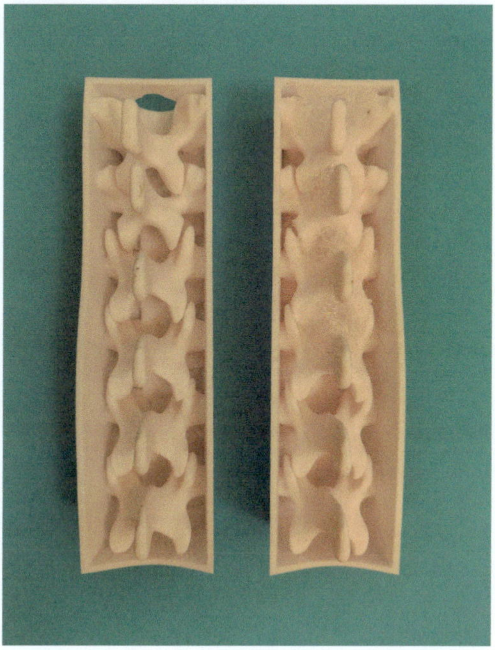

**Fig. 9** The printable epidural module (left) and the silicone layer modeled on the interlaminar foramina to simulate the ligamenta flava (right)

Shape this mixture onto the model. The mixture should be shaped onto the spine until it completely fills the available space, leaving only the most distal surfaces of the spinous processes exposed (Fig. 10).

Allow to dry for 24–48 h.

Once the mixture is dry, if you want to simulate the supraspinous ligament as well, apply a strip of silicone on the supraspinous processes for a thickness of 0.5–1 cm and let it dry for another 24 h.

For connecting the "dural sac" plastic tube and for positioning the silicone skin (all supplied with the simulator), you can easily follow the manufacturer's user manual instructions.

The Epidural Module$^{EESOA}$ is ready to be used (Fig. 11).

The model thus modified, alongside all the features described by the manufacturer, can also be used as an "epiduroscope." By introducing an endoscopic tube (such as the Ambu aScope™ flexible fiberscope) into the prepared channel within the model, the trainee can see in real time the introduction of the epidural needle, the passage of the spinal needle through the epidural needle, and the path of the epidural catheter within the epidural space (Fig. 12).

After having used it for several times, if you feel that the density of the module no longer meets the educational needs, the mixture can be easily removed and reassembled, but usually, the module can be used for a total of about 200–250 punctures. The frequency with which it needs to be changed for each teaching session varies, depending on the amount of water injected by the students during the

**Fig. 10** The printable epidural module (left) and the neoprene layer (right) modeled to simulate the soft tissues

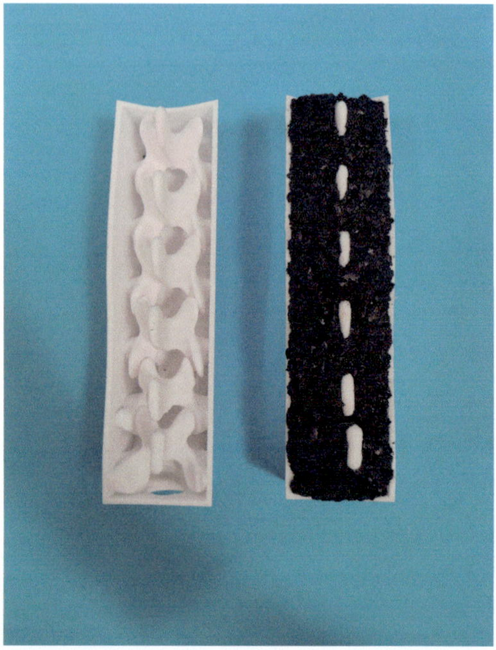

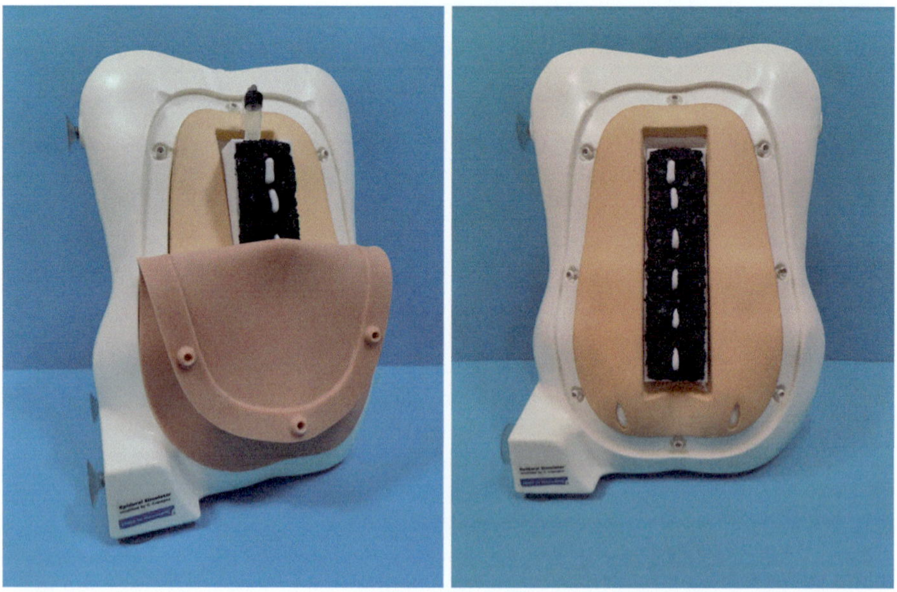

**Fig. 11** The final model inserted into the epidural simulator

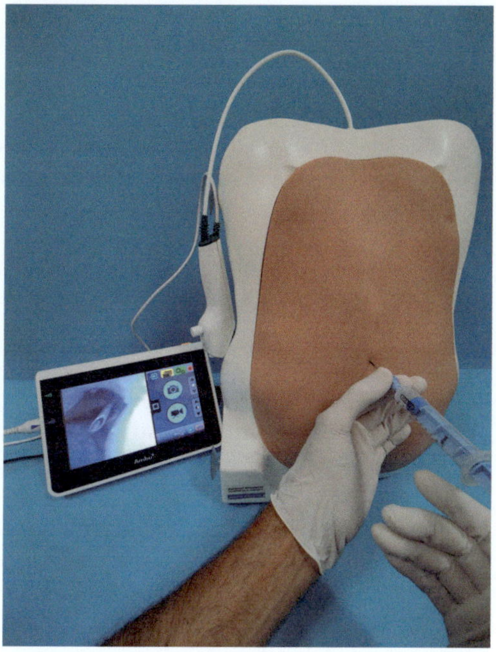

**Fig. 12** Introduction of an endoscopic tube into the prepared channel within the model

procedures, but usually, each module tolerates a teaching session with 2–3 students for a couple of continuous hours of procedure executions.

## 6.3 Realism

The use of a soft mixture allows you to experience the differences in resistance that the operator must learn to appreciate when advancing the Tuohy needle and to differentiate the sensations of false "loss of resistance" as happens when the liquid is injected before reaching the ligamentum flavum.

As in the real patient, the model we designed can also become soaked with water after repeated attempts, making the simulation even more realistic, as the student will find the same sensations of tissue soaking as in reality.

The variable thickness of the "ligamentum flavum" due to the random distribution of silicone (because the silicone is manually modeled on the bone model) will also provide realistically different sensations of resistance in various sectors of the ligament, exactly as it happens in reality.

The presence of a nylon-printed spine model, with real dimensions and consistency, allows the student to experience bone contact on the vertebral arch with and without the ligamentum flavum and to easily learn the maneuvers suitable for solving problems related to this obstacle.

The homogeneity of the materials that are practically glued together without any minimal interruption, unlike the internal modules of commercial simulators that are overlapped and leave a virtual space between the various layers, allows for the realism of the continuous progression of the needle-syringe system, which is difficult to achieve in standard simulators.

Depending on the quantity and quality of the mixture used, modules can be obtained that simulate difficult cases, such as an obese patient (using neoprene fragments with a thickness >2 cm for the mixture) or with a particularly deep epidural space (using a larger amount of mixture).

## 6.4 Validation

In a comprehensive review, Stunt et al. [35] reported that there are, on average, more than 400 medical simulators available on the market for training, but 93.5% of these have not undergone validity testing. Moreover, the main problem with evaluating epidural simulators is that they are usually assessed by Likert-type scales reported by "expert physicians," but due to the subjective nature of this assessment, the results of the studies are often disappointing or controversial [6–8].

The Epidural Module$^{EESOA}$ has been objectively validated by comparing the pressure curves recorded during the advancement of the epidural needle in the tissues of the real patient with those recorded with the simulator [12]. Subsequent studies have confirmed its educational and experimental usefulness [13, 33, 36, 37].

It is currently used routinely for teaching lumbar epidural block in some Italian specialization schools and at the simulation center of the European School of Obstetric Anesthesia.

## References

1. Tuckey J. The epidural potato! Anaesthesia. 1998;53:1232. https://doi.org/10.1046/j.1365-2044.1998.0716h.x.
2. Bromage PR. The epidural potato—and beyond. Anaesthesia. 1999;54:619–20. https://doi.org/10.1046/j.1365-2044.1999.96794ff.x.
3. Leighton BL. A greengrocer's model of the epidural space. Anesthesiology. 1980;70:368–9.
4. Van den Berg A. Teaching Neuraxial analgesia: identification of loss of resistance (epidural) and intrathecal (spinal) placement of needles—avoid "making a lemon" of yourself. Anesth Analg. 2013;117:533–4. https://doi.org/10.1213/ANE.0b013e318296b956.
5. Raj D, Williamson RM, Young D, Russell D. A simple epidural simulator: a blinded study assessing the 'feel' of loss of resistance in four fruits. Eur J Anaesthesiol. 2013;30:405–8. https://doi.org/10.1097/EJA.0b013e328361409c.
6. Uppal V, Kearns R, McGrady E. Evaluation of M43B lumbar puncture simulator-II as a training tool for identification of the epidural space and lumbar puncture. Anaesthesia. 2011;66:493–6. https://doi.org/10.1111/j.1365-2044.2011.06710.x.
7. Lee RA, van Zundert TC, van Koesveld JJ, van Zundert AA, Stolker RJ, Wieringa PA, Gatt SP. Evaluation of the Mediseus epidural simulator. Anaesth Intensive Care. 2012;40:311–8. https://doi.org/10.1177/0310057X1204000215.
8. Pedersen TH, Meuli J, Plazikowski EJ, Buttenberg M, Kleine-Brueggeney M, Seidl C, et al. Loss of resistance: a randomised controlled trial assessing four low-fidelity epidural puncture simulators. Eur J Anaesthesiol. 2017;34:602–8. https://doi.org/10.1097/EJA.0000000000000640.

9. Capogna G, Stirparo S, Caniggia S. Evaluation of a new training device to simulate the epidural and subarachnoid spaces for neuraxial anesthesia techniques. Minerva Anestesiol. 2013;79:385–90.
10. Warrington S, Warrington AM. An inexpensive adult lumbar puncture task-trainer with simulated cerebrospinal fluid. HCA Healthcare J Med. 2020;1:4. https://doi.org/10.36518/2689-0216.1083.
11. Azad M, Montealegre-Gallegos M, Jeganathan J, Yeh L, Hiansen JQ, Meineri M, et al. Low-cost three-dimensional printed phantom for neuraxial anesthesia training: development and comparison to a commercial model. PLoS One. 2018;13:e0191664. https://doi.org/10.1371/journal.pone.0191664.
12. Capogna G, Coccoluto A, Capogna E, Del Vecchio A. Objective evaluation of a new epidural simulator by the CompuFlo® epidural instrument. Anesthesiol Res Pract. 2018;2018:4710263. https://doi.org/10.1155/2018/4710263.
13. Scorzoni M, Gonnella GL, Capogna E, Velardo M, Giuri PP, Ciancia M, et al. Achieving lumbar epidural block competency in inexperienced trainees after a structured epidural teaching model: a randomized, single blind, prospective comparison of CUSUM learning curves. Anesthesiol Res Pract. 2022;2022:1738783. https://doi.org/10.1155/2022/1738783.
14. Odom M, Gomez JR, Danelson KA, Sarwal A. Development of a homemade spinal model for simulation to teach ultrasound guidance for lumbar puncture. Neurocrit Care. 2019;31:550–8. https://doi.org/10.1007/s12028-019-00779-4.
15. Daykin A, Bacon R. An epidural injection simulator. Anaesthesia. 1990;45:235–6. https://doi.org/10.1111/j.1365-2044.1990.tb14694.x.
16. Langton JA, Meiklejohn BH. Pressure generated during insertion of lumbar epidurals: a comparison with the Portex epidural injection simulator. Anaesthesia. 1990;45:1055–6. https://doi.org/10.1111/j.1365-2044.1990.tb14888.x.
17. Stredney D, Sessanna D, McDonald JS, Hiemenz L, Rosenberg LB. A virtual simulation environment for learning epidural anesthesia. In: Weghorst SJ, Sieburg HB, Morgan KS, editors. Medicine meets virtual reality: healthcare in the information age. Amsterdam: IOS Press; 1996. p. 164–75.
18. Bostrom M, Singh SK, Wiley CW. Design of an interactive lumbar puncture simulator with tactile feedback. In: Virtual reality annual international symposium. Proceedings of the IEEE; 1993. p. 280–6.
19. Gorman P, Krummel T, Webster R, Smith M, Hutchens D. A prototype haptic lumbar puncture simulator. In: Medicine meets virtual reality 2000: envisioning healing: interactive technology and the patient–practitioner dialogue; 2000. p. 106–9.
20. Färber M, Hummel F, Gerloff C, Handels H. Virtual reality simulator for the training of lumbar punctures. Methods Inf Med. 2009;48:493–501. https://doi.org/10.3414/ME0566.
21. Lee RA, van Zundert TC, van Koesveld JJ, van Zundert AA, Stolker RJ, Wieringa PA, et al. Evaluation of the Mediseus epidural simulator. Anaesth Intensive Care. 2012;40:311–8. https://doi.org/10.1177/0310057X1204000215.
22. Brazil AL, Conci A, Clua E, Bittencourt LK, Baruque LB, Conci N. Haptic forces and gamification on epidural anesthesia skill gain. Entertain Comput. 2018;25:1–13.
23. Moo-Young J, Weber TM, Kapralos B, Quevedo A, Alam F. Development of Unity simulator for epidural insertion training for replacing current lumbar puncture simulators. Cureus. 2021;13(2):e13409. https://doi.org/10.7759/cureus.13409.
24. Vaughan N, Dubey VN, Wee MYK, Isaacs R. Virtual reality simulation based assessment objectives for epidural training. ASME J Med Devices. 2014;8(2):020948.
25. Senac T, Lelevé A, Moreau R, Krähenbühl L, Sigwalt F, Bauer C. Skill assessment of an epidural anesthesia using the PeriSIM simulator. IEEE Trans Med Robot Bionics. 2021;3:106–14.
26. Regional Anesthesiology and Acute Pain Medicine Fellowship Directors Group. Guidelines for fellowship training in Regional Anesthesiology an doi: 10.1097/AAP.0b013e31820d439f.d Acute Pain Medicine: Second Edition, 2010. Reg Anesth Pain Med. 2011;36(3):282–8.

27. Lorello GR, Cook DA, Johnson RL, Brydges R. Simulation-based training in anaesthesiology: a systematic review and meta-analysis. Br J Anaesth. 2014;112(2):231–45. Epub 2013 Dec 23. https://doi.org/10.1093/bja/aet414.
28. Zendejas B, Brydges R, Wang AT, Cook DA. Patient outcomes in simulation-based medical education: a systematic review. J Gen Intern Med. 2013;28:1078–89. https://doi.org/10.1007/s11606-012-2264-5.
29. Udani AD, Kim TE, Howard SK, Mariano ER. Simulation in teaching regional anesthesia: current perspectives. Local Reg Anesth. 2015;8:33–43. https://doi.org/10.2147/LRA.S68223.
30. Friedman Z, Siddiqui N, Katznelson R, Devito I, Bould MD, Naik V. Clinical impact of epidural anesthesia simulation on short- and long-term learning curve: high- versus low-fidelity model training. Reg Anesth Pain Med. 2009;34:229–32. https://doi.org/10.1097/AAP.0b013e3181a34345.
31. Lim G, Krohner RG, Metro DG, Rosario BL, Jeong JH, Sakai T. Low-fidelity haptic simulation versus mental imagery training for epidural anesthesia technical achievement in novice anesthesiology residents: a randomized comparative study. Anesth Analg. 2016;122(5):1516–23. https://doi.org/10.1213/ANE.0000000000001260.
32. Lydon S, Reid McDermott B, Ryan E, et al. Can simulation-based education and precision teaching improve paediatric trainees' behavioural fluency in performing lumbar puncture? A pilot study. BMC Med Educ. 2019;19:138. https://doi.org/10.1186/s12909-019-1553-7.
33. Capogna E, Coccoluto A, Gibiino G, Del Vecchio A. Compuflo®-assisted training vs conventional training for the identification of the ligamentum Flavum with an epidural simulator: a brief report. Anesthesiol Res Pract. 2019;2019:3804743. https://doi.org/10.1155/2019/3804743.
34. Isaacs E, Wee MYK, Dubey VN, Vaughan N. A survey of trainees' perspectives on epidural training in the United Kingdom. Glob Anesth Perioper Med. 2015;1:121–4. https://doi.org/10.15761/GAPM.1000130.
35. Stunt J, Wulms P, Kerkhoffs G, Dankelman J, van Dijk C, Tuijthof G. How valid are commercially available medical simulators? Adv Med Educ Pract. 2014;14:385–95. https://doi.org/10.2147/AMEP.S63435.
36. Capogna E, Salvi F, Delvino L, Di Giacinto A, Velardo M. Novice and expert Anesthesiologists' eye-tracking metrics during simulated epidural block: a preliminary. Brief observational report. Local Reg Anesth. 2020;13:105–9. https://doi.org/10.2147/LRA.S267879.
37. Capogna E, Coccoluto A, Velardo M. Epidural needle extension through the ligamentum Flavum using the standard versus the CompuFlo®-assisted loss of resistance to saline technique: a simulation study. Anesthesiol Res Pract. 2020;2020:9651627. https://doi.org/10.1155/2020/9651627.

# Assessing Learning

Marco Scorzoni

*There is no effective education without evaluation, because what is not evaluated is devalued [1].*

Over the last decade, the scientific literature has increasingly focused on developing criteria and tools to objectively evaluate procedural skills. This emphasis aims to enhance patient safety by mitigating errors attributed to inadequate training. This chapter underlines the importance of understanding and utilizing each evaluative method for its specific purposes and recognizing its limitations.

The criteria for evaluating doctors in training include direct observation without specific criteria, direct observation with specific criteria (including checklists and global rating scales), psychometric tests, procedural activity logs, and movement analysis. Each of these methods contributes uniquely to the comprehensive evaluation of medical professionals, aligning with the broader goal of ensuring a high standard of clinical competence and patient safety.

## 1 General Principles

Clinical competence cannot be guaranteed by academic qualifications or specialist self-referentiality alone, but requires a standardized and shared scientific reference, such as that expressed by Miller's pyramid [2] (Fig. 1).

M. Scorzoni (✉)
Institute of Anesthesiology and Intensive Care Medicine, Sacro Cuore Catholic University, Rome, Italy
e-mail: marco.scorzoni@policlinicogemelli.it

© The Author(s), under exclusive license to Springer Nature Switzerland AG 2024

G. Capogna (ed.), *How to Teach the Epidural Block in Obstetric Anesthesia*, https://doi.org/10.1007/978-3-031-70211-2_3

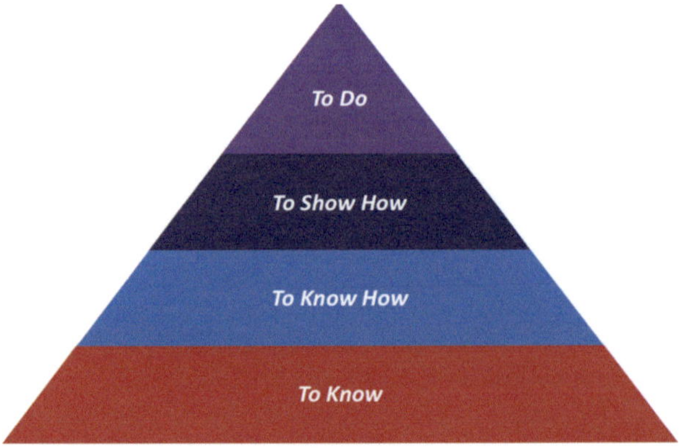


**Fig. 1** Miller's pyramid. (Modified from [2], with permission)

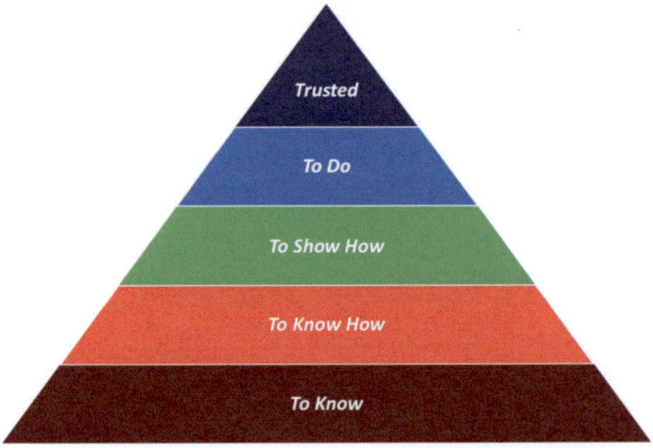


**Fig. 2** Modified Miller's pyramid. (From [3], with permission)

In 1990, psychologist George Miller proposed a reference model that stratified learning into four increasingly complex levels grouped in a virtual pyramid, resulting from the integration of basic knowledge and functional and personal skills with "acted actions" [3]. The first step of this pyramid is "knowing" (To Know): it is built through "formal" learning and through lectures, where the doctor in training acquires the notions and studies the materials necessary to achieve a certain procedural skill. The second step of the pyramid is "knowing how" (To Know How): this level is based on the knowledge of the various steps that, when executed in sequence, allow the studied procedure to be performed. The third step of the pyramid is "showing how" (To Show How): at this point, students repeat the procedure countless times, completely, on the simulator. The last step of the pyramid is "doing" (To Do): the doctors in training find themselves performing the medical procedure in a clinical setting under the supervision of the tutor.

More recently, Miller's pyramid has been modified [3] by adding "trusted" to the apex of the pyramid, meaning having and inspiring trust (Fig. 2). Trust is what the medical trainer places in the doctor in training. This concerns the evaluation of the skills learned and the decision by the tutor that the trainee is now autonomous in performing the learned procedural technique. Trust, therefore, represents the goal of any training course, being linked to the fact that the student can now act without supervision. But this trust also has a second meaning that falls within the behavioral sphere, that is, to inspire trust, as being reliable is one of the crucial characteristics of doctors. Earning trust, being reliable, is not only part of the behavioral characteristics of an individual but requires constant self-awareness, reflection, and attention.

Furthermore, personal, communicative, and relational competence (knowing how to be) must also be added to cognitive competence (knowing) and functional and gestural competence (knowing how to do).

In fact, clinical competence presupposes a balance of the three components in a multidimensional and complex perspective of interaction between the cognitive sphere, clinical decisions, and behavioral attitude. According to Epstein et al. [4], physician competence requires "a thoughtful and judicious use of communication, knowledge, technical skills, clinical reasoning abilities, emotions, and values, the ability to reflect in daily practice, for the benefit of individuals and the community." The "hard skills," the technical skills and abilities, should be integrated with the "soft skills," related to behavioral communication, presentation, and leadership abilities. Clinical competence thus becomes a modus operandi that accompanies and characterizes the professional life of every single doctor [5, 6].

Following Miller's model, it is possible to divide the acquisition of procedural skills and clinical competence into three phases: cognition, integration, and automatism. Cognition is based on understanding the task and the perceptual awareness associated with it and requires a clear description and demonstration of the procedural technique. Integration is achieved when the cognitive phase of the procedural technique is associated with the learning of motor skills for the execution of the technique itself. Finally, when automatism is reached, the procedure becomes mechanical, almost subconscious.

The transition from training in the clinical setting with subjective assessment by a supervisor to a structured program, based on Miller's pyramid with objective evaluation tools, can improve teaching and significantly reduce the incidence of complications during the learning of any medical technique. Direct observation, checklists, evaluation and self-assessment scales, learning curves, and CUSUM curves (see Chapter "Learning Curves") are just some of the tools at our disposal to assess whether the physician in training has reached adequate competence at the third and fourth level of Miller's pyramid [7]. Also, the recording and reviewing of video recordings of procedures performed by trainees can help to get adequate competence in specific procedural skills [8, 9].

## 2 Techniques for Evaluating Learning

Initial evaluation is functional to the detection of the starting knowledge of trainees and is carried out through the administration of specific entrance tests. Evaluation can be eventually formative or summative.

Formative evaluation refers to a series of punctual, analytical, and continuous assessments conducted by tutors during the training process in order to modify teaching and learning activities. Formative assessments, both formal and informal, help both trainees and trainers to improve the learning process while it is taking place and also promote self-assessment of physicians in training. Although assessments generally assign a grade or score, formative assessments provide trainees with feedback which represent important indications for making any corrections to the teaching action and for setting up recovery and/or reinforcement interventions. The objective of formative evaluation, which is personal and not comparative, is to discover the competencies that physicians in training acquire as they move from one learning phase to another.

Summative evaluation is carried out to detect the knowledge and skills of each physician at the end of the learning path. This evaluation also has a formative function because it allows for the last data on trainees' learning to be obtained and provides feedback on the level of their performance at the conclusion of a specific rotation. Summative evaluation also allows for correcting any errors and making the final educational interventions before moving on to another area of content.

Formative evaluation, therefore, supports the learning process in progress, providing information on learning levels so that interventions can be adapted to individual teaching situations and timely corrective strategies can be activated.

Summative evaluation, on the other hand, usually takes place at the end of a learning path and provides, at a specific point in time, evidence of the achievement of the goals set for that training path.

In the various phases, initial, intermediate, and final, the evaluative action is related to the precise identification of the objectives that trainees must achieve.

For the evaluative action to be effective and valid, it requires analysis methods that meet the criteria of reliability, validity, and feasibility. Reliability refers to the degree of consistency of the test between expected data and the results obtained. Validity describes the accuracy of the test, so if it is actually measuring what it set out to measure. Feasibility, finally, refers to the application of the test in the "real world" and its reproducibility [7]. Particular importance is also given to inter-rater reliability, which is the degree of correlation between the scores assigned to the same sample of trainees by two or more independent trainers using the same evaluation tool. Therefore, high inter-rater reliability occurs when the same test, repeated several times on the same trainee by different trainers, provides the same result. This reproducibility varies greatly depending on the complexity of the test and improves with the experience of the trainer physicians, which leads over time to uniformity in the interpretation of the reference standards [7, 10].

In the last decade, scientific literature has increasingly focused on the search for tools, called criteria, that could make the evaluation of procedural skills more objective and valid, in order to make clinical practice safer, protecting patients from "errors" due to inadequate training. Unfortunately, to date, there is no perfect evaluation tool, and therefore, each evaluative test must be used for its purposes, understanding its limitations. The criteria for evaluating doctors in training [7] are as follows: direct observation without specific criteria; direct observation with specific criteria, including checklists and global rating scales; psychometric tests; procedural activity logs; and movement analysis, to which simulation and learning curves, discussed respectively in Chapters "Epidural Simulators" and "Learning Curves", can be added. Reliability, validity, feasibility, and completeness of the main evaluation criteria for learning found in the literature are summarized in Table 1.

## 3 Direct Observation Without Specific Criteria

Direct observation of doctors in training by an expert instructor is a fundamental tool for teaching and evaluating the clinical, procedural, and communication skills of the students. And since the goal of training and evaluation is to make doctors autonomous and therefore able to practice their profession in the clinical environment without the supervision of the tutor, direct observation should be conducted in the clinical setting where trainees must demonstrate their achieved clinical competence [11, 12].

Clinical activity carried out in the field, in a dynamic context, often presents more complex and nuanced aspects than simulation and allows for the evaluation, through direct observation of the trainee on the patient, in the reference clinical setting, of the clinical and behavioral skills required to navigate the complexity of daily medical reality [13].

Directly observing and evaluating students in a clinical setting, in the presence of patients, and subsequently providing feedback, also allows teachers not only to help trainees acquire and improve their clinical–procedural skills but, at the same time, ensures patients maintain high standards of clinical care and safety. Evaluation based on direct observation should, therefore, be an essential component of medical education.

The value of direct participation in clinical activities as a teaching tool is universally recognized by both students and trainer physicians [14–16] as the closer the learning environment is to clinical reality, the more quickly and effectively procedural skills are acquired [17, 18].

Training carried out directly on the patient is perceived by learners as more instructive and exciting than simulation, and moreover, doctors in training, when immersed in everyday clinical reality, show greater enthusiasm for the entire learning process [19].

During direct observation, trainers must continuously model their attitude based on the behavior of the trainees they are observing in order to avoid the Hawthorne effect.

The Hawthorne effect refers to the set of variations, positive or negative, in behavior that occur as a result of the presence of observers, but do not last over time. In the training context, the Hawthorne effect can manifest when trainees change their attitude or performance in response to direct observation by the trainer physician. This can happen either because trainees try to impress the observer or because they feel under pressure to demonstrate that they have reached a certain level of competence.

**Table 1** Reliability, validity, feasibility, and comprehensiveness of techniques to assess technical skills

| Test | Reliability | Validity | Feasibility | Comprehensiveness |
|---|---|---|---|---|
| *Direct observation without criteria* | Poor reliability | Has face validity | Very easy to use | Potentially comprehensive |
| *Checklist* | Excellent reliability in trained observers, especially within the context of an educational study | Intrinsic content validity | Easy to use, requires some training for optimal reliability | Potentially comprehensive: depends on the content of the checklist |
| *GRS* | Excellent reliability in trained observers, especially within the context of an educational study | Construct validity established in anaesthesiology for lumbar epidurals | Easy to use, requires some training for optimal reliability | Potentially comprehensive: depends on the content of the global rating scale |
| *Psychometric testing* | Automated and objective | Limited correlation with early performance in fibreoptic endoscopy | Relatively expensive, requires a degree of expertise to be able to collect, process, and interpret the results | Not comprehensive |
| *Procedural lists* | Self-reported and subject to omissions and inaccuracies | No guarantee that procedures were performed correctly | The easiest form of evaluation | Not comprehensive |
| *Motion analysis* | Objective with a numerical output and so not subject to differences in the opinion of the observer | Construct validity established for epidural anesthesia | Relatively expensive, requires a degree of expertise to be able to collect, process, and interpret the results | Not comprehensive: only evaluates motor skill |

Modified from [7], with permission

To avoid the Hawthorne effect during direct observation, it is important for tutors to be aware of this possibility and adopt appropriate strategies. For example, they can try to create a relaxed and nonjudgmental observation environment, so that trainees feel more at ease and are more likely to show their natural behavior. Medical trainers should also provide authentic and constructive feedback based on the actual performance of the trainees, encouraging them to improve without creating excessive pressure.

The Hawthorne effect highlights the importance of accurate and objective assessment and feedback during direct observation, in order to ensure a truthful evaluation of the skills and competencies acquired by doctors in training [20, 21].

Direct observation is well suited to the field of anesthesiology, where the supervisor–trainee ratio is usually 1:1. Although it is easily implemented in the delivery room and based on the trust relationship between tutor and trainee, direct observation of doctors in training is not always adequately documented. In many cases, evaluation forms used at the end of the rotation in the delivery room are completed by teaching doctors who have not directly observed the trainees. Although remaining a potentially comprehensive assessment tool, direct observation without specific criteria is unfortunately unreliable and invalid and has poor inter-rater reliability [7] (Table 1), and thus, it becomes difficult to decide, solely through direct observation without specific criteria, when the doctor in training is able to perform the lumbar epidural technique independently.

## 4 Direct Observation with Specific Criteria

Direct observation with specific criteria allows for a structured evaluation of the trainee while performing the procedure on the patient.

It investigates not only technical skills but also interaction with patients, colleagues, and professional behavior. Direct observation with specific criteria explores a wide range of competencies, from simple procedures to very complex ones. Moreover, it facilitates the identification of "fragile" doctors in training, individuals who have difficulties in one or more competencies and therefore deserve greater attention and focus of the teacher's training efforts.

Direct observation with specific criteria is, therefore, one of the fundamental cornerstones of training. It is not a simple "prepackaged" tool but represents a "basic attitude" that becomes an integral part of the way of acting in a professional context. There are many criteria-based tools to guide student assessment based on direct observation [22], but tutors, when possible, should use criteria already validated by scientific literature [23]. If specific criteria for a given procedural skill do not exist in the literature, it will be possible to create new ones. The drafting of a new tool for direct observation or the modification of an existing tool always involves compliance with guidelines and must be subjected to validity tests. The tools used for summative assessments will be subjected to a greater number of validity tests compared to the tools used for formative assessments [24]. It is important to emphasize that the validity of a criterion ultimately lies in the medical trainer who uses it and the context in which it is administered. Therefore, it is recommended to devote the right amount of time not only to the design of the criteria but also to the training of the observers who will use them.

The choice of one criterion over another obviously depends on the nature of the assessment, whether quantitative or qualitative.

Regardless of the selected tool, it is important that the criteria provide ample space for analysis and comments [25].

The criteria we will consider for direct observation are checklists and global rating scales.

## 5 Checklists

The birth of the checklist, as we understand it today, can be traced back to a historical event that took place in the distant 1935. On October 30, 1935, the Boeing Model 299, nicknamed "Flying Fortress," lifted off the ground, ready to take flight for the US military aviation test trials. Its competitor in the race, a Douglas DB-1, seemed to have no hope as the Boeing Model carried five times more bombs than required by the army, was faster, and boasted greater autonomy. The Flying Fortress, shortly after takeoff, crashed, exploding upon impact. Two of the five men on board, including the pilot, Major Ployer Hill, lost their lives. The commission awarded the victory to the Douglas project, and Boeing ended up on the brink of bankruptcy. The internal investigation ruled out a mechanical failure and attributed the accident to pilot error. The new airplane, far more complex than its predecessors, required the pilot to simultaneously manage the four engines, retractable landing gear, flaps, trim tabs, and propeller pitch. In performing all these operations, Major Hill had forgotten to disengage the depth and direction rudder locks. The aircraft, in the words of the investigation, had proven "too complex for a human being to fly." A group of expert pilots began to think about how to make the aircraft pilotable. They decided that it was pointless to commission new training programs for Model 299 pilots: it was unlikely that they could accumulate greater knowledge and experience than Hill, the chief test pilot of military aviation. Instead, they had an idea as simple as it was revolutionary: create a checklist (Fig. 3). With the checklist in hand, the pilots continued to fly the Model 299, soon renamed the B-17, which from then on had great success worldwide [26].

In the educational field, checklists can be used during direct observation as specific criteria to evaluate the performance of doctors in training. They divide an activity or technique into several essential components (items) and assign a dichotomous score, such as passed/failed, for each item. Each checklist must be structured and validated for the procedural skill to be assessed and is usually constructed and validated by doctors considered experts in that field [27]. In addition to binary evaluation, within a checklist, it is possible to include more qualitative evaluation items, such as "optimal execution," "sub-optimal execution," and "uncertain execution," which allow for describing how the procedure was performed [9]. One of the main limitations of checklists is that all phases of the procedural skill considered are

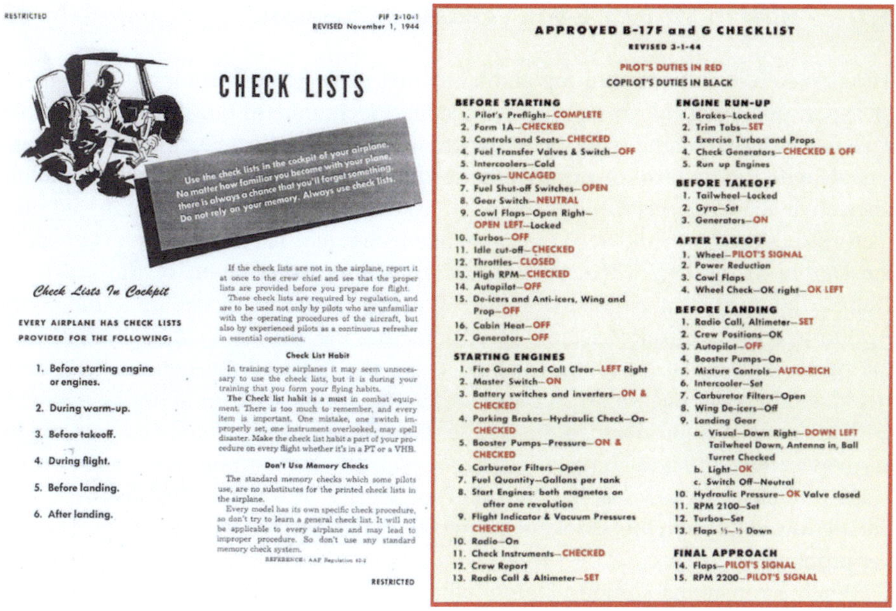

RESTRICTED

PIF 2-10-1
REVISED November 1, 1944

# CHECK LISTS

Use the check lists in the cockpit of your airplane. No matter how familiar you become with your plane, there is always a chance that you'll forget something. Do not rely on your memory. Always use check lists.

*Check Lists In Cockpit*

EVERY AIRPLANE HAS CHECK LISTS PROVIDED FOR THE FOLLOWING:

1. Before starting engine or engines.
2. During warm-up.
3. Before takeoff.
4. During flight.
5. Before landing.
6. After landing.

If the check lists are not in the airplane, report it at once to the crew chief and see that the proper lists are provided before you prepare for flight.

These check lists are required by regulation, and are to be used not only by pilots who are unfamiliar with the operating procedures of the aircraft, but also by experienced pilots as a continuous refresher in essential operations.

**Check List Habit**

In training type airplanes it may seem unnecessary to use the check lists, but it is during your training that you form your flying habits.

**The Check list habit is a must** in combat equipment. There is too much to remember, and every item is important. One mistake, one switch improperly set, one instrument overlooked, may spell disaster. Make the check list habit a part of your procedure on every flight whether it's in a PT or a VHB.

**Don't Use Memory Checks**

The standard memory checks which some pilots use, are no substitutes for the printed check lists in the airplane.

Every model has its own specific check procedure, so don't try to learn a general check list. It will not be applicable to every airplane and may lead to improper procedure. So don't use any standard memory check system.

REFERENCE: AAF Regulation 62-2

RESTRICTED

**APPROVED B-17F and G CHECKLIST**

REVISED 3-1-44

PILOT'S DUTIES IN RED
COPILOT'S DUTIES IN BLACK

**BEFORE STARTING**

1. Pilot's Preflight—COMPLETE
2. Form 1A—CHECKED
3. Controls and Seats—CHECKED
4. Fuel Transfer Valves & Switch—OFF
5. Intercoolers—Cold
6. Gyros—UNCAGED
7. Fuel Shut-off Switches—OPEN
8. Gear Switch—NEUTRAL
9. Cowl Flaps—Open Right—OPEN LEFT—Locked
10. Turbos—OFF
11. Idle cut-off—CHECKED
12. Throttles—CLOSED
13. High RPM—CHECKED
14. Autopilot—OFF
15. De-icers and Anti-icers, Wing and Prop—OFF
16. Cabin Heat—OFF
17. Generators—OFF

**STARTING ENGINES**

1. Fire Guard and Call Clear—LEFT Right
2. Master Switch—ON
3. Battery switches and inverters—ON & CHECKED
4. Parking Brakes—Hydraulic Check—On—CHECKED
5. Booster Pumps—Pressure—ON & CHECKED
6. Carburetor Filters—Open
7. Fuel Quantity—Gallons per tank
8. Start Engines: both magnetos on after one revolution
9. Flight Indicator & Vacuum Pressures CHECKED
10. Radio—On
11. Check Instruments—CHECKED
12. Crew Report
13. Radio Call & Altimeter—SET

**ENGINE RUN-UP**

1. Brakes—Locked
2. Trim Tabs—SET
3. Exercise Turbos and Props
4. Check Generators—CHECKED & OFF
5. Run up Engines

**BEFORE TAKEOFF**

1. Tailwheel—Locked
2. Gyro—Set
3. Generators—ON

**AFTER TAKEOFF**

1. Wheel—PILOT'S SIGNAL
2. Power Reduction
3. Cowl Flaps
4. Wheel Check—OK right—OK LEFT

**BEFORE LANDING**

1. Radio Call, Altimeter—SET
2. Crew Positions—OK
3. Autopilot—OFF
4. Booster Pumps—On
5. Mixture Controls—AUTO-RICH
6. Intercooler—Set
7. Carburetor Filters—Open
8. Wing De-icers—Off
9. Landing Gear
   a. Visual—Down Right—DOWN LEFT Tailwheel Down, Antenna in, Ball Turret Checked
   b. Light—OK
   c. Switch Off—Neutral
10. Hydraulic Pressure—OK Valve closed
11. RPM 2100—Set
12. Turbos—Set
13. Flaps ⅓–½ Down

**FINAL APPROACH**

14. Flaps—PILOT'S SIGNAL
15. RPM 2200—PILOT'S SIGNAL

**Fig. 3** The first checklist

weighted equally, regardless of their actual clinical importance, and thus, a paradox may arise where the trainee can achieve a high score despite being imprecise and omitting important steps of the technique [28]. In clinical practice, for example, by dividing the epidural technique into several equally weighted items, at the end of the evaluation by the tutor, a doctor in training could obtain a high score even if he forgot to adequately prepare the material on the anesthesia cart, did not properly disinfect the patient's skin, or, even worse, did not perform the aspiration test. It is obvious that these three errors do not have the same clinical importance! To overcome this, some phases, considered fundamental for learning a procedural skill, if not performed correctly, can be assessed with a negative score to be subtracted from the overall score. Alternatively, the incorrect execution of a phase could determine the interruption of the procedure itself. Returning to the previous example, the execution of the epidural in the delivery room, trainers can decide whether to associate a negative score with the items they consider fundamental if omitted, for example; whether to remove one point for inadequate preparation of the material on the anesthesia cart; whether to remove one point or two points or even interrupt the procedure for incorrect disinfection of the puncture site; and whether to remove one point or two points or even interrupt the execution of the technique for a failed aspiration test. Maintaining a practical approach, think of the checklist as the recipe for preparing your favorite dish: each step is essential and preparatory to the next, and even a small oversight can affect the final result. Checklists meet the criteria of reliability, validity, and feasibility and have good inter-rater reliability [7, 9] (Table 1), especially if administered by expert tutors trained in evaluation [27].

## 5.1 How to Structure and Validate a Checklist

The first step in fully structuring and validating a checklist is to identify a number of expert doctors in performing the procedural technique in question. The sample selection is based on the criterion of expertise. The aim is to create a pool of professionals with a high level of experience, certified according to the standards of their respective academic institutions, who are asked to define the crucial items to correctly structure the checklist of the examined technique. The second step is to apply the Delphi method [29]. This method refers to the Greek myth of the oracle of Delphi, the most famous oracular center of ancient Greece. According to the myth, Apollo took possession of Delphi after defeating the serpent Python that guarded the place. The oracle of Delphi gained fame and prestige throughout the Greek world and beyond, becoming a point of reference for those seeking divine advice.

The oracle system involved the Pythia, the priestess who acted as an intermediary between Apollo and humans. The Pythia sat above the tripod, positioned over a crack in the earth known as the "navel of the world." It was believed that Apollo's breath flowed through this crack, inspiring the Pythia and allowing her to pronounce her prophecies.

When a consultant came to Delphi with a question or request, various purification rituals were performed. Subsequently, the consultant could ask their question to the oracle. The Pythia, under the influence of the god Apollo, pronounced her prophecies in a cryptic and enigmatic form. Her words were then interpreted by the temple priests, known as "prophets," who translated the prophecies into a more understandable language for the consultant.

The answers of the Delphic oracle had an enormous influence on the political, social, and religious life of ancient Greece. Kings, rulers, generals, and private citizens sought the oracle's advice before undertaking important decisions, such as starting a war or founding a colony. The oracle's answers could influence the choices of leaders and have a significant impact on the historical events of the time. It is important to note that, despite its fame, the Delphic oracle was not considered an infallible source of knowledge. The prophecies were often enigmatic and subject to interpretation. However, the oracle continued to be consulted for centuries, until the final closure of the sanctuary in 393 AD, when Christianity became the dominant religion in the Roman Empire.

The Delphi method indicates, in the scientific community, the modern reinterpretation of the ancient Greek oracle and a new tool for gathering all the useful information to face new and uncertain challenges.

The Delphi method, with its particular structure, allows, through the repeated administration of questionnaires, not only to obtain individual opinions but to raise a "virtual" debate around the object of research among the expert doctors selected to form the sample [30].

The correct and careful application of the Delphi method allows generating the items that will definitively compose our checklist to be created.

It is a qualitative, participatory, and comparative method. Its use is particularly suitable for achieving multiple scientific purposes: comparing several expert doctors belonging to different university/hospital structures, designing the items and the checklist of the procedural skill under investigation, and outlining a probable future development of the technique under study. The "standard" Delphi method is characterized by three phases: an exploratory phase, an analytical phase, and an evaluative phase [31, 32] (Fig. 4).

In the exploratory phase, in strict compliance with international guidelines, the first questionnaire [28, 33] is constructed to be administered to the pool of expert doctors, with a series of questions about the procedural skill to be framed. In this phase, the questions are mostly open and of a general nature, and they aim to bring out points of view that will be refined in the subsequent rounds. This phase aims to focus on the theme, to draw a general picture of the procedural skill to be investigated, which will allow the researchers to precisely outline the concepts, topics, and steps of the technique on which the rest of the research will focus [34]. The analysis of the answers given to the first questionnaire is the last moment of the first phase and the first moment of the second phase, the analytical phase.

The analytical phase is characterized by the construction of a second questionnaire which, in the first part, reports the concepts that emerged from the analysis of the previous one and subsequently addresses in more detail the aspects that emerged in the exploratory phase [35]. In this phase, each expert has the opportunity to find the synthesis of the concepts expressed by the other experts with whom they can compare by commenting and showing their agreement or disagreement. The structure of the Delphi method allows, therefore, the structuring of a communication process among the participants in the group of experts, permitting each to express their knowledge and point of view on a certain procedure, after having known, in an aggregated and anonymous form, the judgment expressed by the others. The results of the analysis of the second questionnaire are directed towards a process of data quantification, and from this originates the evaluative phase that integrates

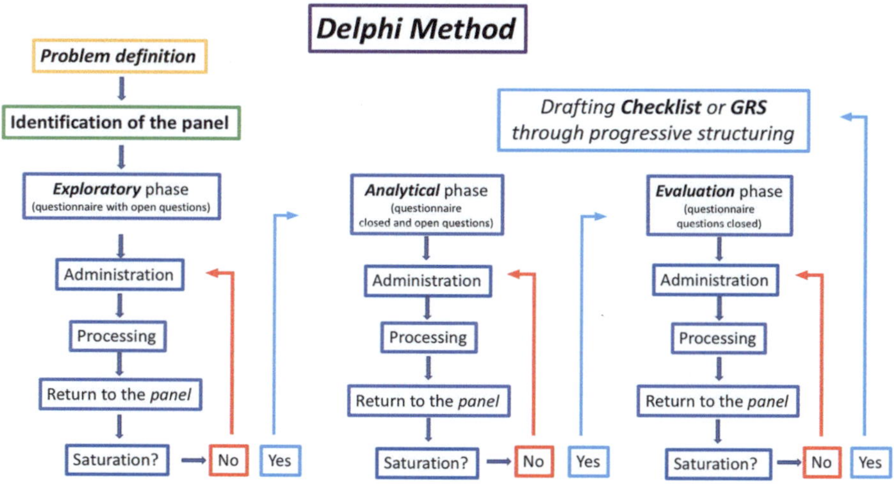


**Fig. 4** Flowchart of the standard Delphi method. (Modified from [32], with permission)

qualitative and quantitative elements [36]. The third and final questionnaire, specific to the evaluative phase, definitively models the items that will make up our checklist and allows each expert to express their judgment regarding the possible future changes to which the procedure under investigation may be subjected.

The Delphi method offers several advantages in its application compared to other methodologies that always assume an exchange of information, a comparison, and group communication, such as conferences and brainstorming. The staged structure of the Delphi method allows a communication process within the group of experts, who can also be geographically distant, in order to facilitate a comparison and mutual exchange of knowledge through self-correction and convergence of individual evaluations, allowed by the feedback process, which also promotes decision-making and intervention problem-solving. Taking place anonymously, this communication process allows for the reduction of leader influence and any psychological and professional barriers: each member is free to express their opinion without fearing the judgment of other participants [37–39]. Finally, the questionnaire gives each physician member of the pool the opportunity to propose new strategies or new problems to submit to the evaluation of others, permitting an evolution of the research methodology. The last positive factor of the Delphi method, always conferred by the phased structure, is the possibility for the team of experts to follow the research of the items in progress in real time, in order to "calibrate" it, if necessary, to new needs. One of the major limitations of this method is certainly the cost of its application, and the success of the methodology is strongly influenced by the quality of the participants in the expert panel [36, 40].

## 5.2 Epidural Checklist

The epidural technique remains an invasive, highly complex anesthesiological procedure, difficult to master as it consists of numerous steps that must be meticulously followed [41, 42]. On the other hand, it represents a fundamental skill in the training curriculum of every anesthetist [43, 44] as it is frequently used in anesthesiological practice and recognized as an integral part of modern obstetrics [45].

Currently, in our university settings, we do not have a standardized and validated method for analyzing the various aspects of epidural catheter placement, let alone for comparing and evaluating the progress of physicians in training in learning this procedural skill. Consequently, trainees often complete their delivery room experience without an objective assessment of their technical abilities related to the epidural block and without having achieved the necessary competence to work independently and safely. Direct observation must, therefore, always be integrated with a system that is as objective as possible and reproducible over time: hence the need to apply the checklist to the epidural technique. In recent years, the scientific literature has begun to produce articles containing epidural checklists, the common goal of which is to standardize the teaching of this difficult-to-learn and insidious procedural skill, making it simple and safe at the same time.

Friedman Z et al. [9] were the first to publish a checklist for the epidural technique (Fig. 5). The idea is that the placement of the epidural catheter represents a relatively complex invasive procedure, consisting of numerous essential technical steps that must be scrupulously followed. The checklist proposed by Friedman consists of 27 items, examined and approved through the Delphi method, by a panel of obstetric anesthetists. The initial item selection is based on a literature review and observation of the most common errors made by physicians in training.

Unfortunately, the limitation of this epidural checklist is that all items have the same weight. We know well that in the clinical reality of the delivery room, not introducing the needle bevel upward, not disinfecting the puncture site correctly, or not performing the aspiration test are actions that have a different impact on the execution of the procedure and the possible onset of complications.

However, to overcome the lack of the quantitative aspect of their evaluation, the same authors of this epidural checklist suggest associating the checklist with a qualitative tool, the global rating scale (see next paragraph). By doing so, the authors have demonstrated a significant correlation between the scores obtained through the epidural checklist and the competence achieved by doctors in training during the learning of the epidural technique, with high inter-rater reliability [9]. According to the authors, this association represents a valid tool for the evaluation of teaching the epidural technique in obstetrics and also allows for calibrating the training on

**Epidural Checklist**

| *Stages Performed* | *Not Performed* | *Performed Poorly* | *Performed Well* |
|---|---|---|---|
| **1.** Ensures patient is positioned comfortably and safely in the middle of the bed | | | |
| **2.** Adjusts height of bed appropriately | | | |
| **3.** Carefully prepares a sterile work surface | | | |
| **4.** Pours antiseptic solution (or has nurse pour it) without contaminating the epidural set | | | |
| **5.** Washes hands and puts on gloves in a sterile fashion | | | |
| **6.** Optimally positions him/herself for the procedure | | | |
| **7.** Prepares the skin at the back widely and aseptically (skin prep 3) | | | |
| **8.** Allows solution to dry | | | |
| **9.** Neatly lays out and prepares all necessary equipment (needles, syringes, local anesthetic) | | | |
| **10.** Asks patient to arch her back | | | |
| **11.** Places drape over patient's back in a sterile fashion | | | |
| **12.** Landmarks site of injection after palpating iliac crests | | | |
| **13.** Warns patient of needle insertion | | | |
| **14.** Infiltrates subcutaneous layers with local anesthetic | | | |
| **15.** Places epidural needle with correct positioning of bevel | | | |
| **16.** Inserts epidural needle through skin, subcutaneous tissue, and into ligament before attaching the syringe | | | |
| **17.** Attaches air/saline filled syringe to the needle hub with needle well controlled | | | |
| **18.** Braces hand/s holding the needle against patient's back in complete control of the needle | | | |
| **19.** Slowly advances needle through supraspinous and interspinous ligaments and into ligamentum flavum while applying pressure on the plunger (continuous or intermittent) | | | |
| **20.** Identifies LOR and immediately releases pressure on the plunger | | | |
| **21.** Notes depth of needle insertion before threading catheter | | | |
| **22.** Warns patient about possible paresthesia during catheter threading | | | |
| **23.** Detaches the syringe and threads the catheter to a depth of 4-5 cm | | | |
| **24.** Pulls the needle out while maintaining correct catheter placement | | | |
| **25.** Carefully aspirates from catheter | | | |
| **26.** Injects test dose through flushed filter | | | |
| **27.** Fixes the epidural catheter securely | | | |

**Fig. 5** An epidural checklist. (From [9], with permission)

fragile trainees, that is, identifying doctors in training who, after a predetermined number of epidurals, have not yet reached adequate competence.

In the literature, there are several articles proposing different models of epidural checklists, all generated with the Delphi method, structured in items grouped into categories. In a study by Flinspach et al. [46], for the first time, an epidural checklist is applied to video tutorials of the epidural technique available on YouTube. The author, starting from the assumption that the modern generation of trainees (Generation Z) is used to using YouTube as a training and consultation tool, examined the tutorials offered by the network that illustrate the epidural technique, having them evaluated by a panel of expert trainers through a structured checklist. Sixteen videos were identified and analyzed. The results of the study are very interesting: (1) only two out of the 16 videos present an epidural technique that almost fully satisfies the administered checklist; (2) standard monitoring and appropriate epidural technique were applied, respectively, only in 42% and 49% of the 16 selected videos; and (3) there is a significant correlation between the duration of the video and the quality of its content. The authors conclude that, since there is no quality control on free digital platforms, it becomes complicated to identify which videos are suitable for educational purposes and that most of the videos on YouTube are not suitable for individual study of the epidural technique due to serious errors and deficiencies concerning patient safety. Flinspach et al. [46] emphasize, once again, the need to structure teaching, even that available on the network, and highlight that checklists, if well structured, represent a versatile tool to be applied even in complex and dispersive contexts, allowing the validation of teaching, even when carried out through the web.

## 6 Global Rating Scales

Global rating scales (GRS) are tools for the systematic recording by the observer of specific qualitative characteristics of the subject analyzed; they are nominal scales and represent a qualitative judgment of what is observed by the examiner.

They can be used as specific criteria during direct observation as they allow guiding and structuring evaluations considering certain procedural skills. GRSs consist of a predetermined set of items, for each of which a qualitative evaluation by the examiner is required. While with checklists, only the presence/absence of a given phenomenon is noted, in a dichotomous way, with global rating scales, an additional element can be added: the observer's evaluation, which allows a classification of the observed parameter [47]. In most cases, a Likert scale is used.

The Likert scale was created in 1932 by American psychologist Rensis Likert, the father of social and organizational psychology. It is presented as a scale, sometimes semi-open, with 3, 5, 7, or 9 elements [48, 49] that define a range of different attitudes or outcomes, from very negative to very positive (Fig. 6). The numerical values on the scale represent the professional judgment of the examiner. Usually, the Likert scale allows for the quantitative measurement of the performance of the subject being examined, through the drafting of a list of statements corresponding

| ***Please answer the following question:*** | | | | | |
|---|---|---|---|---|---|
| ***Likert scale*** | **Very unsatisfied (1)** | **— (2)** | **Neutral (3)** | **— (4)** | **Very satisfied (5)** |
| *Did you find this chapter interesting to read?* | ☐ | ☐ | ☐ | ☐ | ☐ |

**Fig. 6** An example of a semi-open 5-item Likert scale

to a score. In this way, the observer can encode, thanks to standardized judgments, the subject's conduct concerning the procedural skill under examination. To construct Likert scales appropriately, the items, formulated correctly, must be applied to a single topic and composed of descriptive and easily understandable words. Likert scales are widespread, and their use offers several advantages: they allow for an arithmetic and automatic sum of the results; have an intrinsic simplicity of application; are easy-to-understand tools; are simple to analyze based on the attributed responses; are compatible with data quantification techniques; are optimal scales for surveys on specific topics as the data can be examined quickly; are versatile allowing for the analysis of preferences, feelings, points of view, behaviors, and opinions; do not force specific responses; allow for some flexibility; and are appreciated by those who use them.

However, Likert scales have some limitations that are important to consider.

They offer simplified response options, usually a series of statements with a scale of values from "strongly agree" to "strongly disagree." This simplification can reduce the precision and nuance of the responses, limiting the understanding of individuals' true opinions or perceptions.

They do not allow for an in-depth evaluation or a detailed explanation of the responses provided. Trainees may select an option without providing further information on the reason for their choice, which can limit the understanding of the underlying factors influencing their evaluations.

They can lead participants to focus only on a specific aspect of the evaluation, without considering nuances or intermediate elements. This can limit the understanding of more complex or multifaceted opinions.

The questions in Likert scales may be formulated ambiguously or misleadingly, causing confusion or misinterpretations by participants. This could affect the validity of the responses and the overall quality of the data collected.

Finally, Likert scales do not provide a complete or detailed context on the specific circumstances or experiences that influence evaluations. This can limit the understanding of motivations or contextual factors contributing to the responses [50].

GRS are formed by a Likert scale repeated for each item present. The items that make up the GRS are also identified using the Delphi method (Fig. 4).

The application of global rating scales can be extended to the evaluation not only of procedural skills but also of relational and professional abilities.

GRS can be used not only prospectively but also retrospectively to calculate the threshold limit necessary to achieve competence in a particular procedural skill. First, the sum of all the average scores obtained on one's GRS by the doctors in training is calculated and then divided by the total number of students to whom the GRS was administered; the average obtained can be used as a limit score to compare with the arbitrary limit score, which we preset.

It is important to emphasize some of the potential pitfalls that may be encountered when using GRS, such as the "halo" effect. This effect, inherent in the nature of every semi-open GRS, occurs when a positive or negative performance in one item unduly influences the evaluation of performance in other items [51]. For example, in a GRS constructed with a Likert scale from 1 to 5, semi-open (like Friedman's epidural GRS [9]; Fig. 7), if the subject being examined were to fall into score 4, the trainer, if not sufficiently prepared, could be influenced by the evaluation obtained by the trainee in the previous item: assigning a 5 in the wake of a positive halo effect or assigning a 3 in the wake of a negative halo effect. This is a cognitive bias due to the lack of training of evaluators. GRS can also be affected by the "clemency" bias;

| *EPIDURAL GRS* | 1 | 2 | 3 | 4 | 5 |
|---|---|---|---|---|---|
| *Preparation for procedure* | Did not organize equipment well. Has to stop procedure frequently to prepare equipment | | Equipment generally organized. Occasionally has to stop and prepare items | | All equipment neatly organized, prepared, and ready for use |
| *Respect for tissue* | Frequently used unnecessary force on tissue or caused damage | | Careful handling of tissue but occasionally caused inadvertent damage | | Consistently handled tissues appropriately with minimal damage |
| *Time and motion* | Many unnecessary moves | | Efficient time/motion but some unnecessary moves | | Clear economy of movement and maximum efficiency |
| *Instrument handling* | Repeatedly makes tentative or awkward moves with instruments | | Competent use of instruments but occasionally appeared stiff or awkward | | Fluid moves with instruments and no awkwardness |
| *Flow of procedure* | Frequently stopped procedure and seemed unsure of next move | | Demonstrated some forward planning with reasonable progression of procedure | | Obviously planned course of procedure with effortless flow from one move to the next |
| *Knowledge of procedure* | Deficient knowledge | | Knew all important steps of procedure | | Demonstrated familiarity with all aspects of procedure |
| *Overall performance* | Very poor | | Competent | | Clearly superior |

**Fig. 7** Epidural global rating scale (GRS). (From [9], with permission)

evaluators, in fact, if not adequately trained, for fear of penalizing or humiliating trainees through negative judgments, tend to give them a score that is at the high end of the scale, thus affecting the total score. In one study, 95.6% of the scores on a nine-point Likert scale were between 6 and 9.85 [52, 53]. The last bias is represented by the "Pygmalion" effect; this is perhaps the most dangerous effect because it concerns the superficial prejudices that a teacher may have towards their trainee and that influence their evaluative capacity positively or negatively. GRS, therefore, have good reliability and validity and good inter-rater reliability and represent a versatile tool that can be used to evaluate various procedural skills [7, 54].

### 6.1 GRS and Epidural Technique

Global rating scales were first used in the evaluation of teaching the epidural technique in 2006 by Friedman et al. [9] (Fig. 7).

Friedman's GRS consists of six items, selected using the Delphi method and expressed through a semi-open Likert scale ranging from 1 to 5, where 1 represents an insufficient execution in the corresponding item and 5 represents an optimal execution. The six items are the preparation of the procedure, respect for tissues, timing of movements, interaction with materials, fluidity, and knowledge of the steps inherent in the epidural technique. The author adds to his GRS a final item called "overall judgment" in an attempt to make the completion of the form faster, smoother, and therefore suitable for the dynamic reality of the delivery room. Testifying to the versatility of the rating scale he designed, it will be applied in two subsequent studies [44, 55]. The GRS, unlike the checklist, represents a useful tool for evaluating the epidural technique with qualitative criteria, as the Likert scale with values from 1 to 5 guarantees intrinsic objectivity to the method. The limitation of the epidural GRS is that if used by trainers not trained in its administration, it could lose value due to poor inter-rater reliability and suffer from the halo effect. To overcome this, Friedman emphasizes that global rating scales must be used by expert trainers who have previously used the GRS on a homogeneous sample of trainees. Furthermore, by associating the checklist with the GRS, the reliability, validity, feasibility, and inter-rater reliability of the evaluation of the epidural technique can be increased.

The epidural GRS has excellent reliability and good validity when administered by expert trainers, is easy to apply, has high intrinsic inter-rater reliability, and is potentially comprehensive if structured appropriately [7] (Table 1).

## 7 Psychometric Tests

The learning of the epidural technique in obstetrics requires that doctors in training develop new practical skills. According to neurophysiology studies and neuroplasticity processes, a trainee can acquire countless skills during their training, but each specific acquired skill arises from the integration and development of small, fundamental basic skills. Skills are partly inherited, partly acquired, and become, over time and with practice, attitudes that each individual brings to the performances they carry out every day. There are about 50 perceptual–motor skills, ranging from spatial orientation and coordination level to understanding information and manual skills; motor skills provide the necessary information for movement, interaction, and control of the body in the surrounding environment (Table 2) [56, 57].

We are all born with these motor skills, inherent in our species, but some, by nature, are predisposed to develop certain attitudes rather than others; innate motor skills represent both the strength and the limit of one's motor performance [58].

Various psychomotor tests have been proposed in the literature as a tool to select the future orientation of doctors in training (medical specialization oriented to attitudinal skills) and to evaluate the learning of acquired professional skills [57].

The only study that has tried to relate psychomotor tests to the learning of the epidural technique is that of Dashfiel in 2000 [59]. The author subjected ten

**Table 2** Motor abilities according to the literature review

| Motor abilities | Description |
|---|---|
| *Control precision* | Ability to make highly controlled movement adjustments, particularly when large muscle groups are involved |
| *Multi-limb coordination* | Ability to coordinate the movement of several limbs simultaneously |
| *Rate control* | Ability to produce continuous anticipatory movement adjustments in response to changes in the speed of a continuously moving target or object |
| *Arm–hand steadiness* | Ability to make precise arm and hand positioning movements where strength and speed are not required |
| *Finger dexterity* | Ability to manipulate small objects |
| *Manual dexterity* | Ability to manipulate relatively large objects with the hands and arms |
| *Reaction time* | The speed with which an individual can respond, using a prescribed movement, to a stimulus when it appears |
| *Response orientation* | Ability to make quick choices among numerous alternative actions often measured as choice reaction time |
| *Wrist–finger speed* | Ability to rapidly move the wrist and fingers with little or no accuracy demands |
| *Aiming* | A highly restricted type of ability that needs the making of accurate hand movements to targets under speeded conditions |
| *Hand–foot coordination* | Ability to coordinate control of foot movement with hand movement |
| *Hand–eye coordination* | Ability to coordinate control of eye movement with hand movement |
| *Speed of limb movement* | Ability to move arms or legs rapidly but without a reaction time stimulus to reduce movement time |
| *Balance–visual cues* | Ability to maintain total body balance when visual cues are available |
| *Static strength* | Ability to use muscle force to lift, push, pull, or carry objects |
| *Flexibility of movement* | Ability to apply whole-body movement in completing a task by bending, stretching, twisting, or reaching |

Modified from [56], with permission

anesthesia trainees, five men and five women, to two computerized psychometric tests ADTRACK 3 and MAZE, part of the MICROPAT testing system, used in the early 1980s to train US Air Force pilots [60]. After completing the psychometric tests and participating in a structured training program in obstetric anesthesia, the trainees in the study performed their first 50 epidurals. Each procedure performed was recorded in terms of success and failure, and the data obtained were retrospectively evaluated by the same experimenter. The results of the study show a significant correlation between the average failure rate of the epidural technique (incomplete analgesia and/or accidental dural puncture) for the second 25 consecutive epidurals and the score obtained on ADTRACK 3. There is no correlation, however, between the failure rate of the epidural technique and the scores obtained on the MAZE. The author concludes that perceptual/motor skills are not decisive in the initial phase of learning the epidural technique but become decisive after the twenty-fifth procedure performed, allowing the consolidation of the skills acquired in the initial training phase. The perceptual/motor ability represents only one aspect of the epidural technique in obstetric anesthesia and is not sufficient, on its own, in this procedural skill, to achieve clinical competence.

Psychomotor tests are computerized and therefore objective, relatively expensive, have high inter-rater reliability, and at the same time require expert personnel to process and interpret the results, but above all, they are not always exhaustive as they analyze only the perceptual–motor component of the epidural technique [7] (Table 1).

## 8 Self-Assessment and Procedure Registry

Self-assessment can take many forms, including meetings, discussions, moments of reflection, interviews between trainers and trainees, self-assessment tests, and records of activities carried out.

These types of self-assessment have a common denominator: they require doctors in training to honestly review their work in order to establish the skills they have acquired and allow them to identify areas in which they feel less confident. Self-assessment always involves a perception of competence, that is, a subjective judgment, and for this reason, one of the most challenging tasks is to ensure that self-assessment methods also have the levels of quality that are common to all evaluation methods, namely validity, reliability, and feasibility. Self-assessment, therefore, has as its objective the awareness of the doctor in training with respect to the skills possessed and developed during various moments of professional life [61]. Self-assessment also improves communication, as trainees become aware of the areas of the training path in which they have difficulties and are more facilitated in communicating their needs [62]. To become capable self-assessors, trainees must have clear objectives, the ability to develop a clear definition of the procedural skill to be performed, and the ability to independently correct or adjust their training path through constant and timely feedback from the tutor.

Doctors in training do not learn to evaluate their own learning alone, but still need someone to teach them self-verification and self-assessment strategies [63]. Finally, when doctors in training are given the opportunity to suggest how they can be helped in their learning and to indicate which activities or teaching strategies have proven most effective, they become more autonomous and actively involved in the training process [64].

The procedure log (logbook) is the personal training booklet in which the trainee must record all the interventions and procedures performed by them during their training path in order to certify the achievement of educational objectives [65], and it is one of the most common forms of self-assessment of procedural skills due to its low cost and simple application in the clinical setting of the delivery room.

Unfortunately, although it is evident that to progress technically in the execution of the epidural technique, a certain number of epidurals are necessary, the procedure log method is not able to express the number of epidurals needed to achieve clinical competence. The procedure log has clear limitations, especially if used in the summative phase of the evaluation. Lacking close control by the tutor, doctors in training, while thinking they are performing the epidural technique correctly, could make a mistake within the procedure, acquiring a wrong technique and putting the safety of patients in the delivery room at risk [66].

The procedure log is a self-declared evaluation method, subject to omissions and inaccuracies. Moreover, without close monitoring by the training doctors, it does not guarantee that the epidural technique is performed and acquired correctly. Although not complete, it still represents the simplest form of evaluation to implement in the clinical setting of the delivery room [7].

# 9 Other Methods

## 9.1 Movement Analysis

The ICSAD (Imperial College Surgical Assessment Device) is a device designed to analyze hand movements in surgeons [67]. It provides an objective measure of the technical competence achieved in the surgical field, and its use has been introduced in various fields, including anesthesiology [68]. This device uses a tracking system (Isotrak II; Polhemus Inc., Colchester, VT, USA), consisting of an electromagnetic field generator and two 10 mm sensors attached to the back of each hand. A movement analysis software processes the information obtained from the two sensors and calculates the values related to the total distance traveled by each hand, the number of movements made, and the time taken to perform the procedure (Fig. 8). In a study [69], this device is used for the first time as a tool to objectively evaluate the performance of the epidural technique during labor. According to the authors, the use of ICSAD in the evaluation of lumbar epidural technique is based on the assumption that expert anesthetists are able to perform the procedure more efficiently, reducing the overall length expressed in millimeters of hand movements (path length), the total number of movements made, and the time taken. The expert, in fact, has better

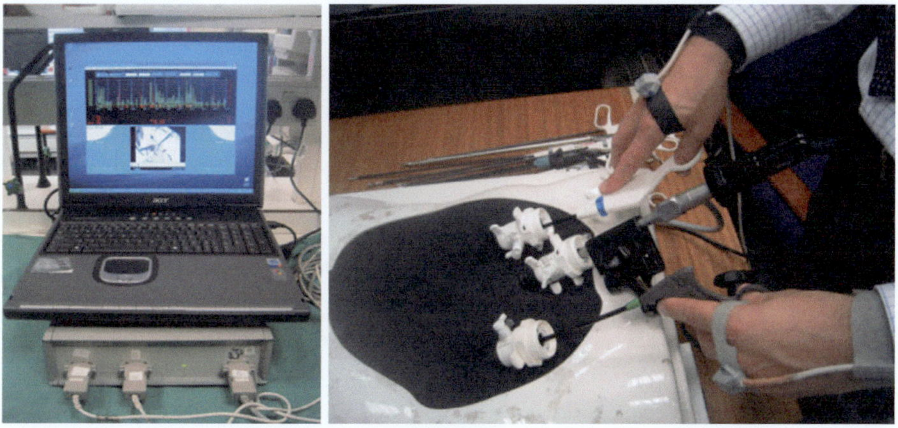

**Fig. 8** The Imperial College Surgical Assessment Device (ICSAD). On the left: a standard laptop with the motion tracking hardware; on the right: the sensors placed on the surgeon's hands for evaluation of a simulated laparoscopic ability. (From [67], with permission)

dexterity, optimizes movements by avoiding oscillations or unnecessary gestures, and performs the technique following the most direct trajectory possible. The trainee, not yet fully understanding the technique, not being fully aware of the critical points that make it up, and not yet having developed adequate mastery of the instruments, should make more movements, cover a greater distance of the hands expressed in mm (path length), and take more time overall in performing the epidural technique compared to the expert. The study compares three groups of doctors: nonexpert residents in the execution of the epidural technique with a number of procedures less than 30, expert residents with a number of procedures greater than 100, and the anesthesiology staff of the delivery room with a number of procedures greater than 500. Through the use of ICSAD, the performance, understood as the number and length of movements and time in the execution of the technique, of the three study groups is examined. The evaluation of the execution of the epidural technique is completed by an epidural checklist associated with an epidural GRS, administered, in a blind manner, to the doctors in the study by a group of expert trainers. The results of the study confirm that the hands of nonexpert residents travel a greater distance, expressed in millimeters (path length), during the execution of the epidural technique, compared to expert residents and the anesthesiology staff of the delivery room. In addition, the novice residents perform more movements and take more time in the execution of the epidural technique compared to the anesthesiology staff of the delivery room (Fig. 9). Nonexpert doctors in training in epidural block, when compared to the anesthesiology staff of the delivery room, obtain significantly lower scores on the GRS and the epidural checklist.

The authors conclude that ICSAD represents a valid tool for reliably measuring competence in performing the epidural technique during labor and is also able to discriminate between different levels of training and experience of the doctors in the study. According to the authors, ICSAD could become, in the future, a fundamental

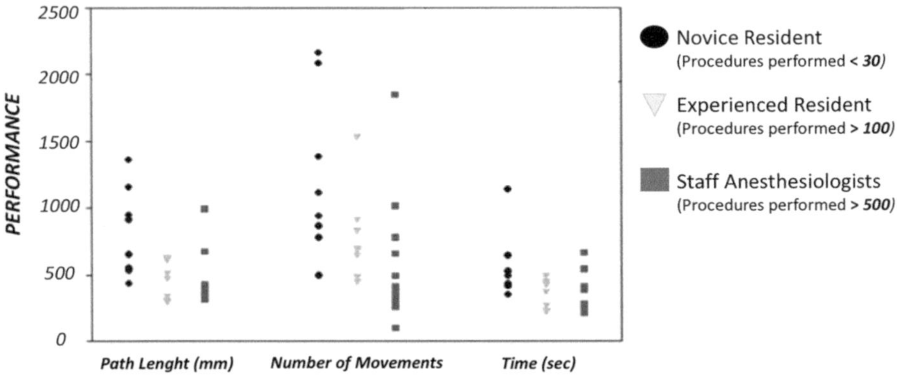


**Fig. 9** ICSAD scores according with the experience level. The number of movements, the length of the path (mm), and the time (s) are reported. (From [69], with permission)

device for evaluating the technical skills acquired for the execution of the epidural technique. However, to make the data derived from ICSAD more complete, it must necessarily be correlated with an epidural checklist or an epidural GRS.

Currently, the limitations of using this method are the relatively high cost, the difficult interpretation of the data that requires adequately trained and educated personnel, and the machine's ability to examine only the motor component and not the entire execution of the epidural technique [7] (Table 1).

## 9.2 Indirect Observation: Video Evaluation

There are certainly significant differences between observing doctors in training directly in the clinical setting and observing their actions indirectly through the acquisition of images recorded on a video medium. Field observation, in fact, represents a unique and engaging experience, which involves an authentic view and can easily be transformed into participatory observation, that is, direct collaboration between the tutor and the doctor in training. However, some aspects of observation may be lost during live participation. Due to its unique characteristic, the live experience is transient and does not always allow the recovery of elements that document and corroborate actions, statements, perceptions, and memories. Moreover, identification can "cloud" the gaze, while problems of time, simultaneity of actions, or complexity of procedural skills under study, such as the epidural technique, can escape direct observation of important details.

Precisely because of its objective value, indirect observation through video can be a valid complementary tool for evaluating and training interns: the method allows for reviewing video sequences, stopping them, or even reworking them by selecting and reassembling images deemed of particular interest for learning the technique. Another positive aspect of video-assisted indirect observation is the sharing of the same training corpus by multiple people, resulting in the standardization of the related procedural skills. The technique, the subject of study, can also be viewed from different perspectives and divided into a certain number of steps, called metrics [70]. In one study [71], indirect observation and metrics were applied to teaching the epidural technique. Seventy-four metrics were structured and validated, identified through 5 rounds by a panel of 3 experts (phase 1), applying the epidural checklist (Fig. 5) and the GRS epidural (Fig. 7) to video-assisted indirect observation of the epidural technique performed by 16 expert and 16 nonexpert physicians (phase 2). The metrics were then applied, using proficiency-based progression (proficiency-based progression, PBP), to a group of nonexpert residents during the execution of the epidural technique on the simulator (phase 3). Proficiency-based progression (PBP) is based on the premise that learning is a gradual process, in which physicians in training acquire and demonstrate specific skills before advancing to more complex levels. In the study, according to the authors, proficiency-based progression implies that trainees advance through a series of 74 metrics described by critical (likely harmful to the patient) and noncritical errors, demonstrating, on the simulator, full understanding of the metric addressed before moving on to the next metric. The goal of proficiency-based progression and the use of metrics described by critical and noncritical errors is to ensure that physicians in training acquire competence in all the steps that make up the technique gradually, with continuous assessment of their abilities and increasing safety for patients. After completing the training period with phase 3, the first ten epidurals performed by the residents in the study were recorded through direct and indirect observation. The results confirm that indirect observation, metrics described through errors, and proficiency-based progression, applied for the first time with an end-to-end process on nonexpert residents in lumbar epidural block, significantly reduce the incidence of failure of the epidural technique in the study group. Moreover, metrics described by errors, if administered by expert trainers, have high validity and high inter-rater reliability (IRR = 0.88) compared to the GRS epidural and the epidural checklist, becoming the ideal tool for evaluating the learning of the lumbar epidural technique. The division into metrics described by critical and noncritical errors, the use of proficiency-based progression, and video-assisted indirect observation are tools recently validated by scientific literature to effectively and objectively structure the teaching of the lumbar epidural technique [71].

A further advantage of video-assisted indirect observation is that it can also focus on the behavior of tutors, which can in turn be analyzed and evaluated by third-party observers.

As for the negative aspects, it is clear that observation is mediated by a tool, and the authenticity of the perception of the educational action can be lost. On the screen, only a part of reality is visible, the one framed, while what has not been captured represents an information gap. In this regard, it is desirable that the material be recorded with one fixed camera, or more than one, maintaining a neutral and always equal point of view, rather than relying on operators who, filming according to their own perspective, would reproduce a subjective perspective.

Furthermore, video-assisted indirect observation is also subject to the Hawthorne effect: those who are filmed generally know they are being filmed, so they may adopt an artificial behavior that does not correspond to reality, unless the use of video has already become an integrated routine in the educational action. Weighing the pros and cons, the positive value of video-assisted indirect observation remains undeniable, especially if seen as preparatory before and as reinforcement during the direct observation of procedural skills.

## 10 The Kirkpatrick Pyramid

The evaluation of training effectiveness should constantly follow the training process. Evaluating learning means identifying the changes that have occurred in individuals' knowledge, skills, and performance as a result of a specific training intervention, in order to ensure coherence between training plans and strategies aimed at achieving certain objectives [72]. The most well-known, appreciated, and used model for evaluating the effectiveness of a training course is undoubtedly the four-level model introduced in 1959 by Donald Kirkpatrick [73, 74] (Fig. 10). This model, revisited in 2016 and named the "New World Kirkpatrick Model" [75–77], is defined as "hierarchical" because each of its evaluation levels is preparatory and therefore necessary for the evaluation of the next level, indicating specific procedures and measurements for each level, suitable for application in any training context, including medical [77].

The four evaluation levels proposed by Kirkpatrick and modified in the "New World Kirkpatrick Model" are reaction, learning, behavior, and results (Fig. 11).

In the reaction, the model aims to detect and measure the satisfaction expressed by participants of a specific training course, regarding educational, organizational, logistical, social, and motivational aspects, including perceptions of usefulness and difficulty of the course itself [78]. The procedural instrument usually used to detect satisfaction parameters is a feedback questionnaire with both closed and open questions, in response to the use of a specific training course. Closed-question feedback questionnaires, composed of Likert scales, are common. The only obstacle to this first phase of detection is often the negligence of participants in completing

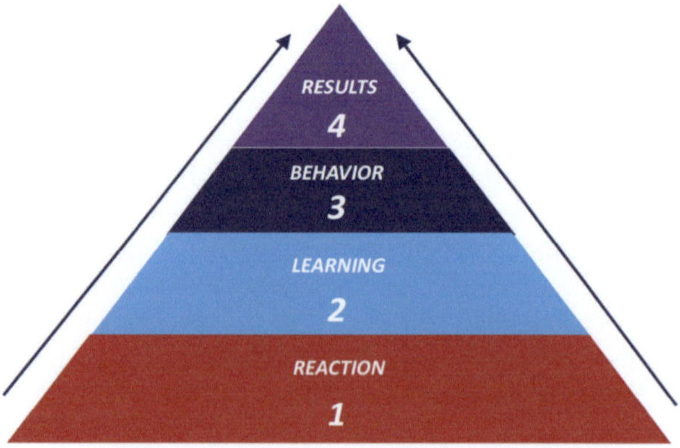


**Fig. 10** Kirkpatrick's model. (From [74], with permission)

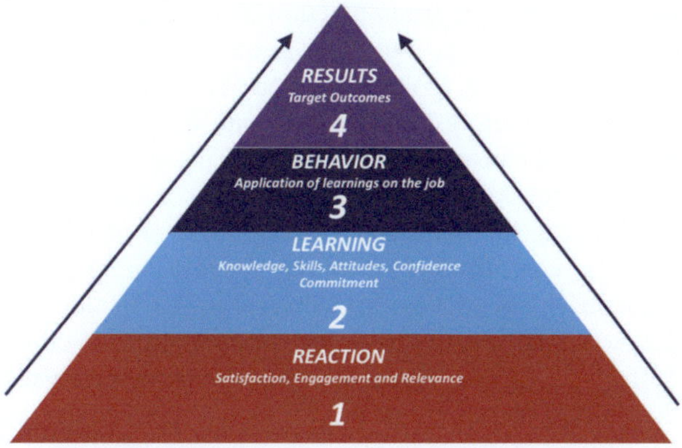


**Fig. 11** New World Kirkpatrick Model. (Modified from [75], with permission)

feedback questionnaires presented at the end of the course. The participant may perceive this questionnaire more as a waste of time than as an important moment for organizational and, indirectly, personal improvement.

The second level, learning, is objective compared to the subjectivity expressed in the evaluations of satisfaction and appreciation of the previous level.

The purpose of this level is to measure and detect the actual educational effectiveness of the training course in terms of knowledge retention and improvement of individual skills and performance. Generally, tests are administered before the training course (pre-test or pre-assessment) and at the end of the course itself (post-course or end-of-course test). The questions of the two tests are homologous, in order to measure the achievement of the predetermined learning objectives as objectively as possible.

The third level, behavior, arises from the need to measure and quantify the actual application in the clinical setting of the new knowledge acquired in a specific training course [74]. Learning, in fact, to bring tangible benefits, must be applied in daily activities and work: the goal of training is not simply the growth of the individual, but of the organization as a whole for patient safety.

It should be noted that high satisfaction and a high level of learning do not always result in a high level of transfer in the clinical field [79]. This transfer is influenced by many factors not calculated and considered in the previous two levels, such as the support and assistance given to participants at the end of a training course, especially by tutors and direct supervisors of the doctor in training. In this case, measurement techniques consist of administering evaluation tests before the training intervention and several months later, using detection techniques and judgment scales to detect purely behavioral aspects [80].

The fourth level, results, is related to the outcomes produced by effective training. In the medical field, the last level evaluates whether learning is transferred into daily practice, improving clinical practice and ensuring greater patient safety [78, 81].

Despite the considerable success of Kirkpatrick's model, it has some significant limitations [76]: (1) the model places evaluation at the end of the training process, minimizing the feedback function for each level; (2) it is a result-oriented model and does not take into account the various environmental and individual factors that can influence training; (3) the expected objectives in level 3 and level 4, the most important at the training level, are difficult to evaluate in clinical practice; and (4) the hierarchical cause–effect relationship between objectives and positive results of the training process is only partially true: favorable reactions contribute to greater learning, leading to changes in behavior and positive program results; however, good learning can also go through uncomfortable and frustrating phases. Finally, Kirkpatrick's model assumes that the higher the level reached by doctors in training, the more important the training result obtained in clinical reality. But the evaluation of the training path cannot be separated from the objective of the training. If, in fact, the training path aims to improve the knowledge of a specific procedural skill and has a purely notional purpose, then the results of level 1, reaction, will represent our objective. If the evaluation aims, instead, to measure the achievement of clinical competence, we will pay attention to the results of level 3, behavior.

Despite its limitations, Kirkpatrick's model is used by the World Health Organization (WHO) as a guide for evaluating training [82].

*To teach is to learn twice. (Joseph Joubert).*

## References

1. Padula MS, Aggazzotti G, D'Ambrosio G. Come insegnare la medicina generale. 1st ed. Athena Audiovisuals; 2015.
2. Cruess RL, Cruess SR, Steinert Y. Amending Miller's pyramid to include professional identity formation. Acad Med. 2016;91:180–5. https://doi.org/10.1097/ACM.0000000000000913.
3. Ten Cate O, Carraccio C, Damodaran A, Gofton W, Hamstra SJ, Hart DE, et al. Entrustment decision making: extending Miller's pyramid. Acad Med. 2021;96:199–204. https://doi.org/10.1097/ACM.0000000000003800.
4. Epstein RM, Hundert EM. Defining and assessing professional competence. JAMA. 2002;287:226–35. https://doi.org/10.1001/jama.287.2.226.
5. Medical Professionalism Project. Medical professionalism in the new millennium: a physicians' charter. Lancet. 2002;359:520–2. https://doi.org/10.1016/S0140-6736(02)07684-5.
6. Tay KT, Ng S, Hee JM, Chia EWY, Vythilingam D, Ong YT, et al. Assessing professionalism in medicine—a scoping review of assessment tools from 1990 to 2018. J Med Educ Curric Dev. 2020;7:2382120520955159. https://doi.org/10.1177/2382120520955159.
7. Bould MD, Crabtree NA, Naik VN. Assessment of procedural skills in anaesthesia. Br J Anaesth. 2009;103:472–83. https://doi.org/10.1093/bja/aep241.
8. Swartz MH, Colliver JA, Bardes CL, Charon R, Fried ED, Moroff S. Global ratings of videotaped performance versus global ratings of actions recorded on checklists: a criterion for performance assessment with standardized patients. Acad Med. 1999;74:1028–32. https://doi.org/10.1097/00001888-199909000-00018.
9. Friedman Z, Katznelson R, Devito I, Siddiqui M, Chan V. Objective assessment of manual skills and proficiency in performing epidural anesthesia-video-assisted validation. Reg Anesth Pain Med. 2006;3:304–10. https://doi.org/10.1016/j.rapm.2006.04.006.
10. Chuan A, Wan AS, Royse CF, Forrest K. Competency-based assessment tools for regional anaesthesia: a narrative review. Br J Anaesth. 2018;120:264–73. https://doi.org/10.1016/j.bja.2017.09.007.

11. Kogan JR, Hatala R, Hauer KE, Holmboe E. Guidelines: the do's, don'ts and don't knows of direct observation of clinical skills in medical education. Perspect Med Educ. 2017;6:286–305. https://doi.org/10.1007/s40037-017-0376-7.
12. Walton M, Barraclough B. Clinical supervisors: are they the key to making care safer? BMJ Qual Saf. 2013;22:609–12. https://doi.org/10.1136/bmjqs-2012-001637.
13. Eva KW, Bordage G, Campbell C, Galbraith R, Ginsburg S, Holmboe E, Regehr G. Towards a program of assessment for health professionals: from training into practice. Adv Health Sci Educ Theory Pract. 2016;21:897–913. https://doi.org/10.1007/s10459-015-9653-6.
14. Teunissen PW, Scheele F, Scherpbier AJ, van der Vleuten CP, Boor K, van Luijk SJ, et al. How residents learn: qualitative evidence for the pivotal role of clinical activities. Med Educ. 2007;41:763–70. https://doi.org/10.1111/j.1365-2923.2007.02778.x.
15. Teunissen PW, Boor K, Scherpbier AJ, van der Vleuten CP, van Diemen-Steenvoorde JA, van Luijk SJ, et al. Attending doctors' perspectives on how residents learn. Med Educ. 2007;41:1050–8. https://doi.org/10.1111/j.1365-2923.2007.02858.x.
16. Watling C, Driessen E, van der Vleuten CP, Lingard L. Learning from clinical work: the roles of learning cues and credibility judgements. Med Educ. 2012;46:192–200. https://doi.org/10.1111/j.1365-2923.2011.04126.x.
17. Kneebone R, Nestel D, Wetzel C, Black S, Jacklin R, Aggarwal R, et al. The human face of simulation: patient-focused simulation training. Acad Med. 2006;81:919–24. https://doi.org/10.1097/01.ACM.0000238323.73623.c2.
18. Lane C, Rollnick S. The use of simulated patients and role-play in communication skills training: a review of the literature to august 2005. Patient Educ Couns. 2007;67:13–20. https://doi.org/10.1016/j.pec.2007.02.011.
19. Bokken L, Rethans JJ, van Heurn L, Duvivier R, Scherpbier A, van der Vleuten C. Students' views on the use of real patients and simulated patients in undergraduate medical education. Acad Med. 2009;84:958–63. https://doi.org/10.1097/ACM.0b013e3181a814a3.
20. LaDonna KA, Hatala R, Lingard L, Voyer S, Watling C. Staging a performance: learners' perceptions about direct observation during residency. Med Educ. 2017;51:498–510. https://doi.org/10.1111/medu.13232.
21. Paradis E, Sutkin G. Beyond a good story: from Hawthorne effect to reactivity in health professions education research. Med Educ. 2017;51:31–9. https://doi.org/10.1111/medu.13122.
22. Kogan JR, Holmboe ES, Hauer KE. Tools for direct observation and assessment of clinical skills of medical trainees: a systematic review. JAMA. 2009;302:1316–26. https://doi.org/10.1001/jama.2009.1365.
23. Hauer KE, Holmboe ES, Kogan JR. Twelve tips for implementing tools for direct observation of medical trainees' clinical skills during patient encounters. Med Teach. 2011;33:27–33. https://doi.org/10.3109/0142159X.2010.507710.
24. Artino AR Jr, La Rochelle JS, Dezee KJ, Gehlbach H. Developing questionnaires for educational research: AMEE guide no. 87. Med Teach. 2014;36:463–74. https://doi.org/10.3109/0142159X.2014.889814.
25. Daelmans HE, Mak-van der Vossen MC, Croiset G, Kusurkar RA. What difficulties do faculty members face when conducting workplace-based assessments in undergraduate clerkships? Int J Med Educ. 2016;7:19–24. https://doi.org/10.5116/ijme.5689.3c7f.
26. Boyne WJ. The checklist. Air Force Mag. 2013;96:52–6.
27. Naik VN, Perlas A, Chandra DB, Chung DY, Chan VW. An assessment tool for brachial plexus regional anesthesia performance: establishing construct validity and reliability. Reg Anesth Pain Med. 2007;32:41–5. https://doi.org/10.1016/j.rapm.2006.10.009.
28. McKinley RK, Strand J, Ward L, Gray T, Alun-Jones T, Miller H. Checklists for assessment and certification of clinical procedural skills omit essential competencies: a systematic review. Med Educ. 2008;42:338–49. https://doi.org/10.1111/j.1365-2923.2007.02970.x.
29. Khurana MP, Raaschou-Pedersen DE, Kurtzhals J, Bardram JE, Ostrowski SR, Bundgaard JS. Digital health competencies in medical school education: a scoping review and Delphi method study. BMC Med Educ. 2022;22:129. https://doi.org/10.1186/s12909-022-03163-7.

30. Humphrey-Murto S, Varpio L, Wood TJ, Gonsalves C, Ufholz LA, Mascioli K, et al. The use of the Delphi and other consensus group methods in medical education research: a review. Acad Med. 2017;92:1491–8. https://doi.org/10.1097/ACM.0000000000001812.
31. Green P, Edwards EJ, Tower M. Core procedural skills competencies and the maintenance of procedural skills for medical students: a Delphi study. BMC Med Educ. 2022;22:259. https://doi.org/10.1186/s12909-022-03323-9.
32. Habibi A, Sarafrazi A, Izadyar S. Delphi technique theoretical framework in qualitative research. Int J Eng Sci. 2014;3:8–13.
33. Goff BA, Nielsen PE, Lentz GM, Chow GE, Chalmers RW, Fenner D, et al. Surgical skills assessment: a blinded examination of obstetrics and gynecology residents. Am J Obstet Gynecol. 2002;186:613–7. https://doi.org/10.1067/mob.2002.122145.
34. Hartman N, Wittler M, Askew K, Manthey D. Delphi method validation of a procedural performance checklist for insertion of an ultrasound-guided internal jugular central line. Am J Med Qual. 2016;31:81–5. https://doi.org/10.1177/1062860614549762.
35. Ahlin C, Löfmark A, Klang-Söderkvist B, Johansson E. Development of instruments for assessment of knowledge and skills in performing venepuncture and inserting peripheral venous catheters. J Vasc Access. 2013;14:364–72. https://doi.org/10.5301/jva.5000147.
36. Romero-Collado A. Essential elements to elaborate a study with the (e)Delphi method. Enferm Intensiva. 2021;32:100–4. https://doi.org/10.1016/j.enfi.2020.09.001.
37. de Villiers MR, de Villiers PJ, Kent AP. The Delphi technique in health sciences education research. Med Teach. 2005;27:639–43. https://doi.org/10.1080/13611260500069947.
38. Taylor E. We agree, don't We? The Delphi method for health environments research. HERD. 2020;13:11–23. https://doi.org/10.1177/1937586719887709.
39. Barrett D, Heale R. What are Delphi studies? Evid Based Nurs. 2020;23:68–9. https://doi.org/10.1136/ebnurs-2020-103303.
40. Varndell W, Fry M, Lutze M, Elliott D. Use of the Delphi method to generate guidance in emergency nursing practice: a systematic review. Int Emerg Nurs. 2021;56:100867. https://doi.org/10.1016/j.ienj.2020.100867.
41. Kopacz DJ, Neal JM, Pollock JE. The regional anesthesia "learning curve". What is the minimum number of epidural and spinal blocks to reach consistency? Reg Anesth. 1996;21:182–90.
42. Konrad C, Schüpfer G, Wietlisbach M, Gerber H. Learning manual skills in anesthesiology: is there a recommended number of cases for anesthetic procedures? Anesth Analg. 1998;86:635–9. https://doi.org/10.1097/00000539-199803000-00037.
43. Birnbach DJ, Santos AC, Bourlier RA, Meadows WE, Datta S, Stein DJ, et al. The effectiveness of video technology as an adjunct to teach and evaluate epidural anesthesia performance skills. Anesthesiology. 2002;96:5–9. https://doi.org/10.1097/00000542-200201000-00007.
44. Friedman Z, Siddiqui N, Katznelson R, Devito I, Bould MD, Naik V. Clinical impact of epidural anesthesia simulation on short- and long-term learning curve: high- versus low-fidelity model training. Reg Anesth Pain Med. 2009;34:229–32. https://doi.org/10.1097/AAP.0b013e3181a34345.
45. Hawkins JL. Epidural analgesia for labor and delivery. N Engl J Med. 2010;362:1503–10. https://doi.org/10.1056/NEJMct0909254.
46. Flinspach AN, Raimann FJ, Schalk R, Bepler L, Ruesseler M, Flinspach MH, et al. Epidural catheterization in obstetrics: a checklist-based video assessment of free available video material. J Clin Med. 2022;11:1726. https://doi.org/10.3390/jcm11061726.
47. Vassiliou MC, Feldman LS, Andrew CG, Bergman S, Leffondré K, Stanbridge D, Fried GM. A global assessment tool for evaluation of intraoperative laparoscopic skills. Am J Surg. 2005;190:107–13. https://doi.org/10.1016/j.amjsurg.2005.04.004.
48. Likert R. A technique for the measurement of attitude scales. Arch Psychol. 1932;22:1–55.
49. Zoller A, Hölle T, Wepler M, Radermacher P, Nussbaum BL. Development of a novel global rating scale for objective structured assessment of technical skills in an emergency medical simulation training. BMC Med Educ. 2021;21:184. https://doi.org/10.1186/s12909-021-02580-4.
50. Svensson E. Construction of a single global scale for multi-item assessments of the same variable. Stat Med. 2001;20:3831–46. https://doi.org/10.1002/sim.1148.

51. Holbrook MB. Using a structural model of halo effect to assess perceptual distortion due to affective overtones. J Consum Res. 1983;10:247–52. https://doi.org/10.1086/208963.
52. Holmboe ES, Hawkins RE. Methods for evaluating the clinical competence of residents in internal medicine: a review. Ann Intern Med. 1998;129:42–8. https://doi.org/10.7326/0003-4819-129-1-199807010-00011.
53. Thompson WG, Lipkin M Jr, Gilbert DA, Guzzo RA, Roberson L. Evaluating evaluation: assessment of the American Board of Internal Medicine Resident Evaluation Form. J Gen Intern Med. 1990;5:214–7. https://doi.org/10.1007/BF02600537.
54. Ma IW, Zalunardo N, Pachev G, Beran T, Brown M, Hatala R, et al. Comparing the use of global rating scale with checklists for the assessment of central venous catheterization skills using simulation. Adv Health Sci Educ Theory Pract. 2012;17:457–70. https://doi.org/10.1007/s10459-011-9322-3.
55. Hayter MA, Friedman Z, Katznelson R, Hanlon JG, Borges B, Naik VN. Effect of sleep deprivation on labour epidural catheter placement. Br J Anaesth. 2010;104:619–27. https://doi.org/10.1093/bja/aeq063.
56. Toale C, Morris M, Ryan DM, Boland F, Doherty EM, Traynor OJ, et al. Baseline assessments of psychomotor aptitude are associated with the future operative performance of surgical trainees a prospective observational cohort study. Ann Surg. 2022;278:148. https://doi.org/10.1097/SLA.0000000000005565.
57. Changiz T, Amouzeshi Z, Najimi A, Adibi P. A narrative review of psychomotor abilities in medical sciences: definition, categorization, tests, and training. J Res Med Sci. 2021;26:69. https://doi.org/10.4103/jrms.JRMS_965_19.
58. Dashfield AK, Smith JE. Correlating fibreoptic nasotracheal endoscopy performance and psychomotor aptitude. Br J Anaesth. 1998;81:687–91. https://doi.org/10.1093/bja/81.5.687.
59. Dashfield AK, Coghill JC, Langton JA. Correlating obstetric epidural anaesthesia performance and psychomotor aptitude. Anaesthesia. 2000;55:744–9. https://doi.org/10.1046/j.1365-2044.2000.01419.x.
60. Bartam D. The development of an automated testing system for pilot selection: the MICROPAT project. Appl Psychol Int Rev. 1987;36:279–98.
61. Yates N, Gough S, Brazil V. Self-assessment: with all its limitations, why are we still measuring and teaching it? Lessons from a scoping review. Med Teach. 2022;44:1296–302. https://doi.org/10.1080/0142159X.2022.2093704.
62. Colliver JA, Verhulst SJ, Barrows HS. Self-assessment in medical practice: a further concern about the conventional research paradigm. Teach Learn Med. 2005;17:200–1. https://doi.org/10.1207/s15328015tlm1703_1.
63. Raghoebar-Krieger HM, Sleijfer D, Bender W, Stewart RE, Popping R. The reliability of logbook data of medical students: an estimation of interobserver agreement, sensitivity and specificity. Med Educ. 2001;35:624–31. https://doi.org/10.1046/j.1365-2923.2001.00963.x.
64. Ward M, Gruppen L, Regehr G. Measuring self-assessment: current state of the art. Adv Health Sci Educ Theory Pract. 2002;7:63–80. https://doi.org/10.1023/a:1014585522084.
65. Straker TM, Metz S. An innovative use of an online procedure logbook to improve airway training among anesthesiology residents. J Educ Perioper Med. 2014;16:E074.
66. Assessment of technical skills. In: Nuefeld VR, Norman GR, editors. Assessing clinical competence. New York: Springer; 1985. p. 259–74.
67. Aggarwal R, Moorthy K, Darzi A. Laparoscopic skills training and assessment. Br J Surg. 2004;91:1549–58. https://doi.org/10.1002/bjs.4816.
68. Corvetto MA, Fuentes C, Araneda A, Achurra P, Miranda P, Viviani P, et al. Validation of the imperial college surgical assessment device for spinal anesthesia. BMC Anesthesiol. 2017;17:131. https://doi.org/10.1186/s12871-017-0422-3.
69. Hayter MA, Friedman Z, Bould MD, Hanlon JG, Katznelson R, Borges B, et al. Validation of the Imperial college surgical assessment device (ICSAD) for labour epidural placement. Can J Anaesth. 2009;56:419–26. https://doi.org/10.1007/s12630-009-9090-1.
70. Gallagher AG. Metric-based simulation training to proficiency in medical education: what it is and how to do it. Ulster Med J. 2012;81:107–13.

71. Kallidaikurichi Srinivasan K, Gallagher A, O'Brien N, Sudir V, Barrett N, O'Connor R, et al. Proficiency-based progression training: an 'end to end' model for decreasing error applied to achievement of effective epidural analgesia during labour: a randomised control study. BMJ Open. 2018;8:e020099. https://doi.org/10.1136/bmjopen-2017-020099.
72. Mansouri M, Lockyer J. A meta-analysis of continuing medical education effectiveness. J Contin Educ Health Prof. 2007;27:6–15. https://doi.org/10.1002/chp.88.
73. Kirkpatrick DL. Evaluation of training. In: Craig RL, editor. Training and development handbook: a guide to human resource development. New York: McGraw Hill; 1976. p. 301–19.
74. Johnston S, Coyer FM, Nash R. Kirkpatrick's evaluation of simulation and debriefing in health care education: a systematic review. J Nurs Educ. 2018;5:393–8. https://doi.org/10.3928/01484834-20180618-03.
75. Liao S, Hsu S. Evaluating a continuing medical education program: new world Kirkpatrick model approach. Int J Manag Econ Soc Sci. 2019;8(4):266–79.
76. Allen LM, Hay M, Palermo C. Evaluation in health professions education-is measuring outcomes enough? Med Educ. 2022;56:127–36. https://doi.org/10.1111/medu.14654.
77. Kirkpatrick JD, Kirkpatrick WK. Kirkpatrick's four levels of training evaluation. Alexandria (VA): ATD press. Yardley S, Dornan T. 2012. Kirkpatrick's levels and education 'evidence'. Med Educ. 2016;46:97–106.
78. Parker K. A better hammer in a better toolbox: considerations for the future of programme evaluation. Med Educ. 2013;47:440–2. https://doi.org/10.1111/medu.12185.
79. Parker K, Burrows G, Nash H, Rosenblum ND. Going beyond Kirkpatrick in evaluating a clinician scientist program: it's not "if it works" but "how it works". Acad Med. 2011;86:1389–96. https://doi.org/10.1097/ACM.0b013e31823053f3.
80. Reeves S, Zwarenstein M, Goldman J, Barr H, Freeth D, Hammick M, et al. Interprofessional education: effects on professional practice and health care outcomes. Cochrane Database Syst Rev. 2008;(1):CD002213. https://doi.org/10.1002/14651858.CD002213.pub2.
81. Moreau KA. Has the new Kirkpatrick generation built a better hammer for our evaluation toolbox? Med Teach. 2017;39:999–1001. https://doi.org/10.1080/0142159X.2017.1337874.
82. World Health Organization. Evaluating training in WHO. WHO/– HSE/GIP/ITP/2011.2. Geneva: World Health Organization; 2010.

# Learning Curves

Gian Luigi Gonnella

Although many of the variables that influence the outcome of medical procedures (such as lumbar epidural blocks) to be learned cannot be included in the model that defines the learning curve, the use of a curve to show the progress of learning a particular task over time is the most practical way to describe how quickly the operator's performance is improving. The analysis of LC-CUSUM (learning curve-cumulative sum technique) can be used to assess competence in practical procedures in the medical field by establishing an acceptable and unacceptable failure rate at the beginning of the process, providing a clear graphic representation of the trend of outcomes of a series of consecutive procedures (epidural blocks) performed over time. Despite some limitations, CUSUM analysis is a powerful tool for the evaluation of medical staff performance, allowing for timely corrections and/or improvements.

## 1 History and Definition

In 1936, Wright, an aeronautical engineer, hypothesized that the productive efficiency of any activity continuously increases as the activity is repeated and proposed a mathematical function to describe the effect of learning on the production costs of the aerospace industry [1].

In the industrial field, the quantification of the efficiency of a given performance is often evident, but in medicine, it is more difficult to assess the practical skills of an operator.

G. L. Gonnella (✉)
Institute of Anesthesiology and Intensive Care Medicine, Sacro Cuore Catholic University, Rome, Italy
e-mail: gianluigi.gonnella@gmail.com

© The Author(s), under exclusive license to Springer Nature Switzerland AG 2024

G. Capogna (ed.), *How to Teach the Epidural Block in Obstetric Anesthesia*,
https://doi.org/10.1007/978-3-031-70211-2_4

To measure the learning of a technique (such as anesthesia, for example), we can evaluate two factors: one related to the anesthesia procedure and the other related to the patient's outcome.

The results related to the procedure itself are generally easier to analyze and therefore more commonly used, even if they are only indirectly linked to the patients' outcomes. There has been a recognized need for tools that provide objective results, useful for evaluating a physician's performance in performing a medical procedure, and multidimensional charts that take into account all significant variables and are therefore suitable for providing a more accurate representation of learning a specific operation.

## 2 Construction of the Learning Curve

The underlying theory of the learning curve assumes that the efficiency of those learning a task improves over time in direct proportion to the number of times they perform that task. This concept can be graphically represented (Fig. 1).

The original model for determining a learning curve uses the formula $Y = aX^b$, where $Y$ is the average time on the measured duration; a represents the time taken to perform the first attempt; $X$ represents the total number of completed attempts made; and b represents the slope of the learning curve.

The formula predicts that the more attempts made, the less time is needed to learn a given task (Fig. 2). The formula can be used to predict the learning of a simple task by a student or help companies predict the production rate of a product, as theorized by Wright.

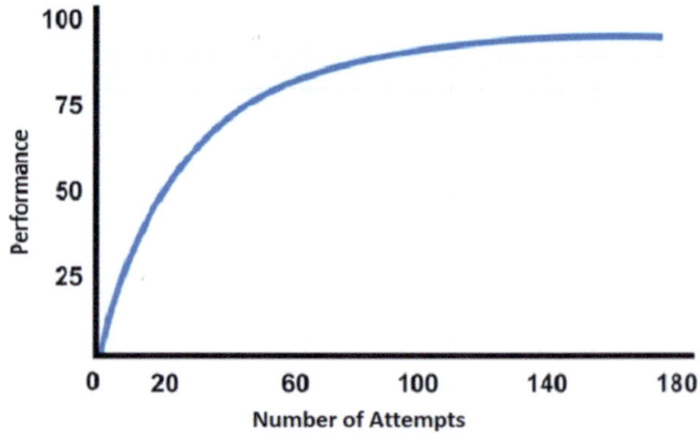


**Fig. 1** Graphical correlation between performance and number of attempts. As the number of attempts increases, there is an improvement in performance

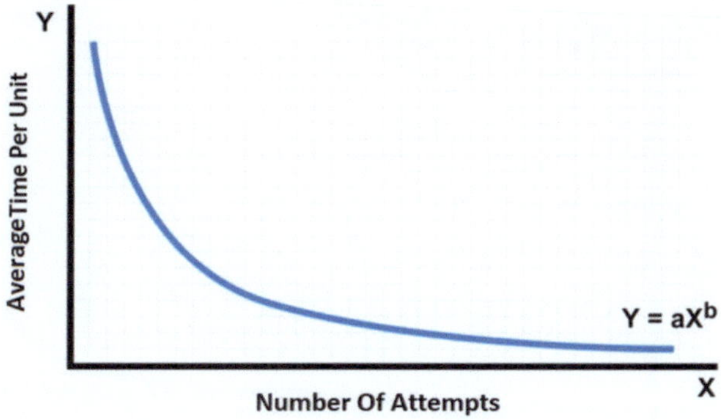


**Fig. 2** Representation of the cumulative average model or "Wright's model." The more attempts made, the less time is needed to learn a given task

## 3 Example of a Complex Learning Curve

Although the theory states that, in general, more attempts correspond to a reduction in the time needed for learning, it does not always work this way. Many factors can influence the final results, resulting in a variety of different learning curve shapes. In Fig. 3, a complex curve is described, representing a substantial synthesis of the different curves. The beginning of the curve indicates that learning is initially slow. The second phase of the curve shows an increase, indicating that the learner is consolidating his/her skills in performing this technique. The third phase of the curve indicates a plateau during which the student feels he has learned the technique. The fourth phase of the curve shows that the student is still improving the skill. The fifth and final phase of the curve represents the point where the skill becomes automatic, often referred to as "overlearning."

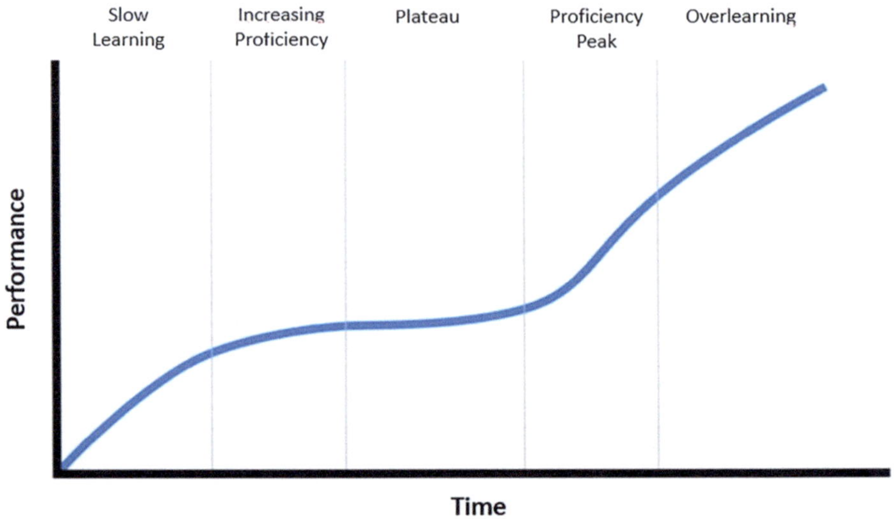


**Fig. 3** Representation of a complex learning curve. At the beginning of the curve, the learning process is initially slow. The second phase of the curve shows an increase (the learner is consolidating his/her skills) in performing this technique. The third phase of the curve indicates a plateau during which the student feels he has learned the technique. The fourth phase of the curve shows that the student is still improving. The fifth phase of the curve represents the point where the skill becomes automatic

## 4 Examples of Applications of Learning Curves

Many of the variables that influence the outcome of the procedure to be learned cannot be included in the model that defines the learning curve. Let us take the example of learning to read. In this field of application, variables could include phonetics, vocabulary, type of reading material, teaching methods, motivation, prior knowledge, and much more. The learning curve model requires that a variable be traceable over time and that it be measurable and repeatable. Individual motivation, for example, would be difficult to measure. Therefore, learning to read is a complex procedure involving many variables and is not ideal for constructing a learning curve.

Monitoring the learning curve is most commonly used in organizational/industrial management to improve production through improving workforce performance. In other words, as the worker learns to operate a production machine by following procedural steps, they become faster and more competent in using it, reducing production costs. Suppose a product takes 2 h to make; such a product could theoretically be put on the market at a price that reflects this production duration. But what would happen if around the fiftieth time that product was made, the production times were reduced to 1 h? It would probably happen that it would be on the market at a higher price (based on longer labor costs and times) and consequently would sell less. Therefore, in the industrial field, the learning curve can be used to predict and plan potential costs when production performance changes.

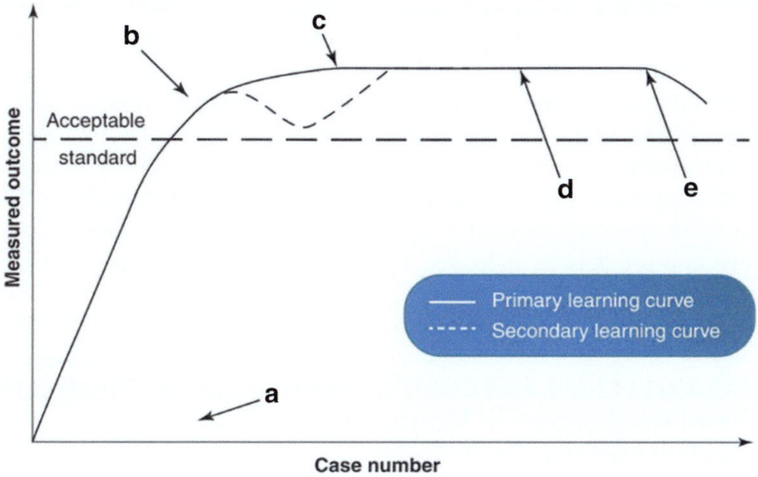


**Fig. 4** Phases of a hypothetical learning curve. (A) Beginning of training; (B) the procedure can be performed independently and competently; (C) additional experience slightly improves results; (D) the plateau is reached; (E) reduction in performance level (advancement of age, deterioration of manual dexterity, vision, memory). The alternative curve (dashed line between B and C) shows a temporary deterioration in performance after achieving technical competence. (Adapted from [2] with permission)

Learning curves also find practical application in the medical field. For example, in the operating room, many of the tasks performed by a surgeon are repetitive, allowing the use of a curve to show the progress of learning a particular performance over time.

A hypothetical graph of a learning curve is illustrated in Fig. 4, showing four main phases.

The starting point A represents the beginning of training. The second phase, identified by a growing curve (we can identify this phase on the graph in the curve between point A and point B), describes how quickly the operator's performance is improving as they learn and master a complex procedure.

Improvements in terms of performance tend to be faster at first and then taper off, as the degree of improvement achieved with each attempt decreases as the technique becomes more refined.

In the third phase, the operator reaches an adequate execution standard, and the procedure can be done independently and competently (point B). Additional experience can slightly improve the results (point C), until reaching a plateau (point D). In the fourth phase, with advancing age, manual dexterity, vision, memory, and cognitive abilities may deteriorate, which can outweigh any advantage derived from long experience, leading to a drop in performance level (point E). An alternative curve (dashed line) can also be drawn, showing a temporary deterioration in performance after achieving technical competence. The postulated reasons for this temporary curve dip are the effect of dealing with more difficult cases or excessive confidence in one's abilities, resulting in technical or judgment errors [2].

The trend just described can be applied to learning the epidural technique, and the curve that describes its progression is one of the most common tools for assessing how the doctor in training is progressing in this skill. As already mentioned, this curve is generated by tracking success or failure relative to the number of attempts. Using this method, Kopacz et al. [3] demonstrated that it takes about 20–25 epidural or spinal procedures to achieve adequate competence, but if a 90% success rate is desired, 45–60 attempts at epidural anesthesia are required. This study has formally established the minimum number of epidural blocks needed for a doctor in training to achieve competence, as indicated by the Accreditation Council for Graduate Medical Education (ACGME).

## 5 Control Chart and CUSUM Learning Curve: Construction and Application in Monitoring the Learning of the Epidural Technique

The CUSUM (cumulative sum technique) analysis originates from a statistical tool developed in the economic field with the purpose of monitoring the quality of production processes, called the control chart. A production process is characterized by variability, which can be divided into natural variability, intrinsic to the process, and variability caused by external sources. The variability introduced by external factors is the subject of control, is higher than the natural variability, and can lead a production line to produce defective items. A process with variability caused by external factors is said to be out of control.

The control chart is the most reliable tool for determining whether a process is still under control or out of control. It is a graphical representation that shows the values of the control statistic alongside a central line (central line, CL) representing the nominal value of that statistic when the process is under control, an upper control line (up control limit, UCL) representing the highest acceptable value that the statistic can assume if the process is under control, and a lower control line (low

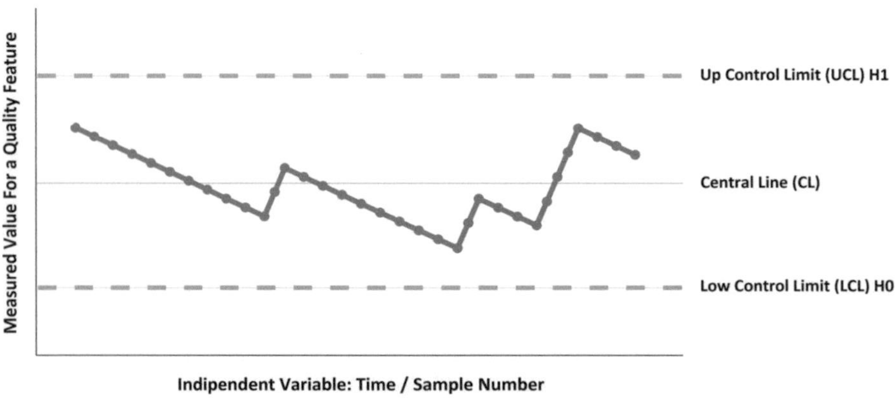


**Fig. 5** Control chart: graphical representation of a process under control

control limit, LCL) representing the lowest acceptable value that the statistic can assume if the process is under control (Fig. 5).

The statistic we are interested in, and from which the respective control chart takes its name, is the CUSUM (cumulative sum) statistic, which has "memory," meaning a statistic that takes into account its previous values and is therefore preferable to others for detecting small process variations.

The control statistic $w(t)$ of the CUSUM curve is thus a cumulative measure of the deviations of the variable representing a specific attribute of a production process at time $t$ ($xt$) from the average of the same values recorded in the reference period ($x1, x2, \ldots, xt$). The general formula for w(t) can be expressed as:

$$w(t) = \max\left[0, w(t-1) + (xt - \mu - k)\right]$$

where $w\ (t - 1)$ is the value of w at time $(t - 1)$, $\mu$ is the reference average, and $k$ is a slope coefficient of the curve.

The idea behind the CUSUM curve represented in control charts is to monitor the value of $w(t)$ concerning the threshold values identified by the previously described LCL and UCL, beyond which the process that has undergone a significant deviation from the average is considered out of control. In this case, a corrective action can be taken to bring the process back to normal "functioning" levels.

Thus, indicating with $w(t)$ the control statistic at time t as a function of measurements of characteristic X, the following hypothesis system of the type is verified:

H0: $w(t) \in$ (LCL, UCL).
H1: $w(t) \neq$ (LCL, UCL).

Accepting the null hypothesis, the process is considered under control, meaning that no control statistic values exceed the aforementioned lower and upper limits; otherwise, at the first observation of the alternative hypothesis H1, an alarm is triggered on the possible out-of-control process.

This control statistic is a function of the characteristic being controlled. There are different types of functions, and the choice depends on the type of variable to be monitored within a production process (dimensions, number of pieces, etc.).

Replacing the concept of quality with that of performance, defined earlier based on learning (understood as improvement following repetitions), and using a statistic with memory (CUSUM) to describe this performance, there will be a process that will certainly increase over time because, as observed with learning curves, a task repeated several times will require less time for each subsequent repetition.

The objective, therefore, will no longer be to keep the process under control (i.e., accept the null hypothesis) but to observe its passage beyond the upper and lower limits, interpreting it respectively as performance not under control, and therefore not safe, or an improvement in performance.

The analysis of LC-CUSUM (learning curve-cumulative sum technique) can be used to assess competence in practical procedures in the medical field by establishing an acceptable and unacceptable failure rate at the beginning of the process. A

CUSUM chart is a graphical representation of the trend of outcomes of a series of consecutive procedures performed over time. On the y-axis, the value of the CUSUM statistic is represented, and on the x-axis, the number of consecutive attempts is represented. Before starting a CUSUM monitoring scheme, some design decisions need to be made. First, it is necessary to establish:

- Acceptable (p0) and unacceptable (p1) failure rates, which are determined through expert discussion.
- Probabilities of type I and II errors (α: false-positive errors; β: false-negative errors).

From these parameters, the upper limit H1 and the lower limit H0 are estimated, beyond which the value of the CUSUM statistic will indicate a change in performance.

The null hypothesis to be tested is that the actual failure rate is not different from the acceptable failure rate. If the CUSUM curve exceeds the upper decision limit (H1) from below, the failure rate is significantly higher than the acceptable failure rate. If the CUSUM curve exceeds the lower decision limit (H0) from above, the actual failure rate does not differ significantly from the acceptable failure rate with the probability of a type II error (Fig. 6).

The variables of the LC-CUSUM curve are always binary. For example, in the case of the epidural block [4], a score can be assigned with a value equal to 0 to indicate a "success" and a value equal to 1 to indicate a "failure." The epidural block is considered a success (score = 0) when the procedure is completed without any intervention from the tutor or other staff member and if the epidural block provided effective analgesia. Conversely, it is defined as a "failure" (score = 1) when at least one of the following conditions occurs: (a) the epidural procedure was completed with assistance from another staff member; (b) when the instructor decided, after interrupting the procedure performed by the trainee, to perform the procedure himself; and (c) when the epidural block produced ineffective analgesia.

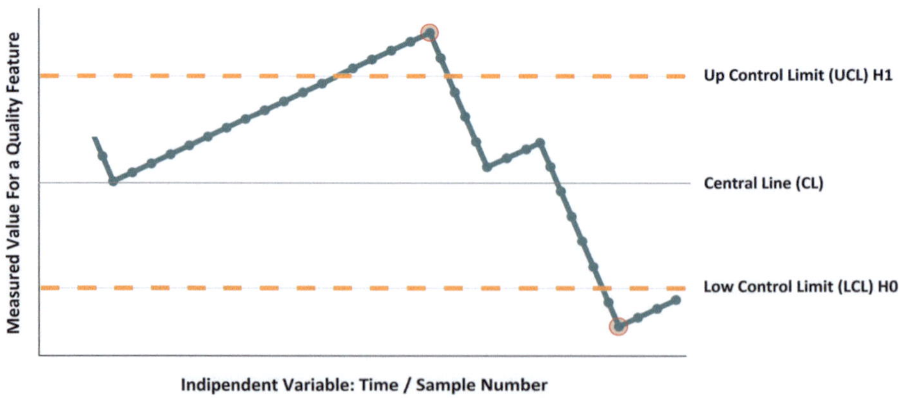


**Fig. 6** The CUSUM curve exceeds the upper decision limit (H1) from below and (H0) from above (points highlighted by the red circle). It means that the process is out of control

Starting from point 0, the LC-CUSUM curve will decrease with each success and increase with each failure, thus describing an improvement in performance each time the LC-CUSUM curve crosses the lower limit (Fig. 6).

If the curve remains between two boundary lines, the results are indeterminate, and the null hypothesis cannot be accepted or rejected, and further observations are needed.

Competence is achieved when the graphical trend falls below two adjacent boundary lines calculated at H0, 2H0, 3H0, and 4H0. Competence is lost, instead, if the chart rises and crosses two calculated boundary lines.

An experienced physician should have a CUSUM learning curve that indicates the continuous maintenance of competence, while a physician in training should have an increasing CUSUM learning curve. The slope of the curve is a measure of progress in learning the new skill: the greater the slope, the slower the progress. When the curve eventually flattens (no slope), this indicates that the new skill has been learned. However, CUSUM analysis is a statistical method that investigates the outcome rather than the process of performing a procedural skill. The LC-CUSUM curve allows the observer to decide whether a learning process (of the epidural technique) is under control or has become out of control, at which point the process needs to be stopped, as the quality has decreased below acceptable limits.

Starting from the concepts just mentioned, Fig. 7 shows an example of interpreting the performance trend of three medical trainees in our delivery room who performed 45 consecutive lumbar epidural blocks. It can be observed that the trainee

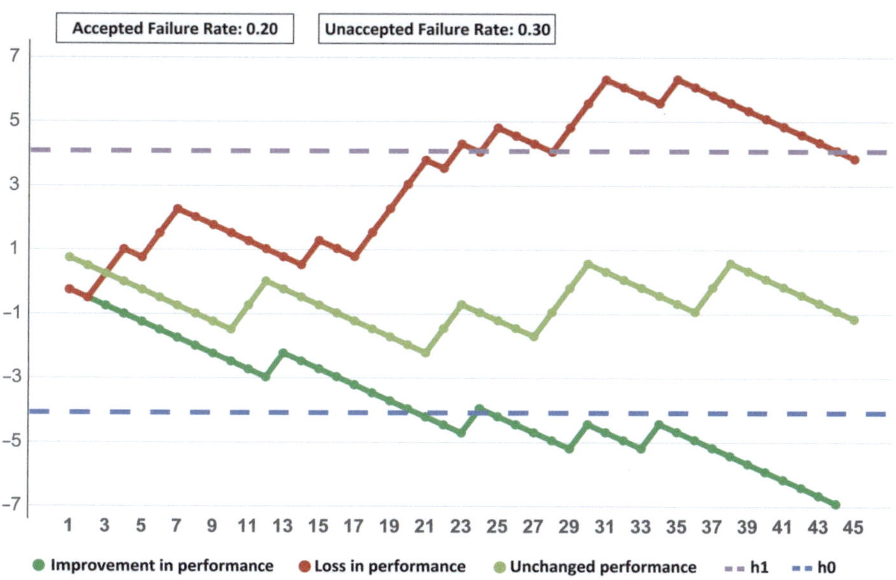


**Fig. 7** Interpretation of CUSUM curves applied to performance trends in 45 consecutive epidural blocks of three trainee doctors: trainee doctor represented in red shows a decline in performance; trainee doctor indicated in dark green shows a progressive improvement in performance; trainee doctor indicated in light green shows no change in performance

identified with the dark green color showed an improvement in performance from the beginning, reaching full mastery (competence) of the procedure at attempt number 20 (where the curve meets the lower dashed boundary line, H0). A completely different performance trend from the previous one is represented by the trainee indicated by the red color, who from the third attempt shows a worsening until the twenty-third epidural where it crosses the upper boundary line H1, which represents the lack of competence in the procedure and more precisely an out-of-control performance trend. The performance trend of the light green trainee, remaining within the two upper and lower boundary lines (H1 and H0), does not show substantial performance changes. Using CUSUM charts, the average number of epidurals needed to achieve competence for inexperienced novices can vary significantly from 46 to 77, depending on the definition used for "success" [5].

We believe that an Institution which is responsible for a specific training should accurately define what is the acceptable and unacceptable failure rate during the learning of the lumbar epidural block as well as other anesthesia procedures. In this sense, the use of the LC-CUSUM curve provides valid support for monitoring the path of those learning a new skill and, indirectly, the abilities of those teaching such a skill.

By reducing the acceptable and unacceptable failure rates to 0.10 and 0.25, it can be seen in Fig. 8 how the same three doctors show different performance trends

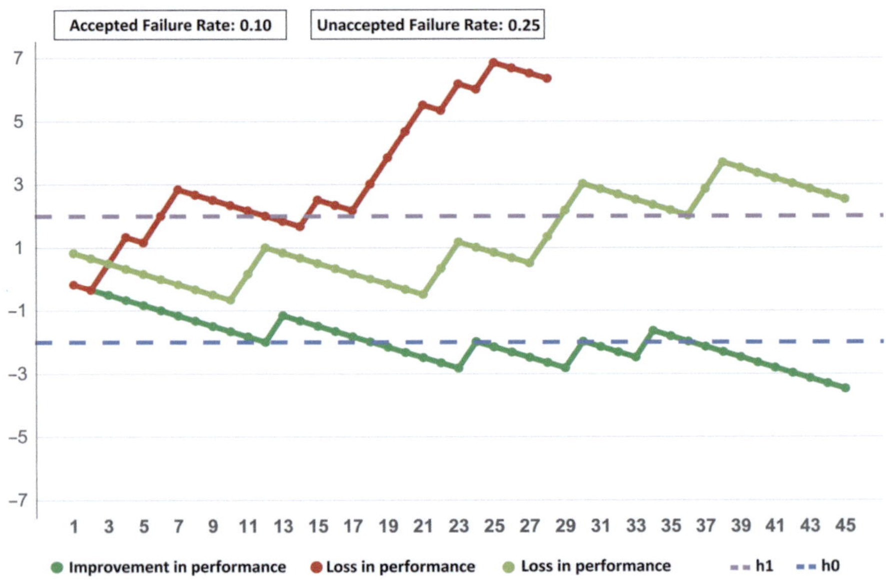


**Fig. 8** Performance variations due to changes in acceptable and unacceptable failure rates compared to those used in the graphs of Figs.6 and 7. It can be observed how the light green trainee, who in the previous chart did not show performance changes, demonstrates a worsening of the performance trend starting from the twenty-ninth epidural, where it crosses the $h_l$ control line, upon reducing the acceptable and unacceptable failure rates

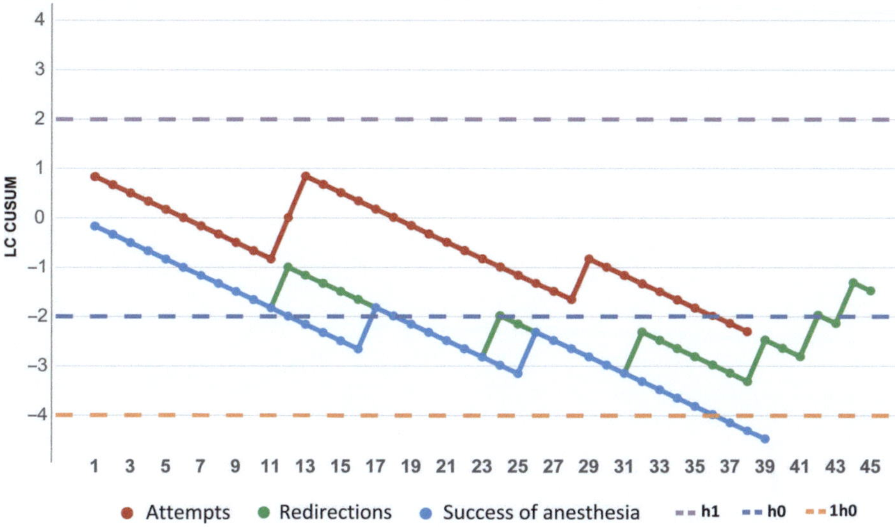


**Fig. 9** The LC CUSUM curve analyzing epidural block performance: number of attempts, redirections, and anesthesia success. These three skills are depicted with the colors red, green, and blue, respectively. The same individual gets competence in different moments for each skill

from those of the previous chart with higher failure rates. In particular, it can be observed that the light green trainee, who in the previous chart did not show performance changes, demonstrates a worsening of the performance trend starting from the twenty-ninth epidural, where it crosses the H1 control line, upon reducing the acceptable and unacceptable failure rates.

This shows that using different failure rates can produce different results, determining a change in the average number of procedures needed to achieve competence, and this could create confusion and inconsistency in the interpretation of CUSUM analysis. It is indeed known that setting different acceptable and unacceptable failure rates can produce different results and therefore different interpretations of the LC-CUSUM curve [6].

The LC CUSUM curve can be used to analyze epidural block performance observing one subject for the progression of several skills (Fig. 9) such as the number of attempts (number of times the Tuohy needle is completely retracted and reinserted from and into the skin before finding the epidural space), the number of redirections (number of trajectory changes without completely retracting the needle from the skin before finding the epidural space), and the number of times the epidural block results in an anesthesia success (decrease in pain from uterine contraction). It can be observed that it took different times for the same subject to reach competence in different skills (number of attempts, redirection, success of anesthesia). The crossing with $h_0$ in fact was obtained at the eleventh, eighteenth, and thirty-sixth epidural blocks, respectively. In the example shown in Fig. 10 in the whole period of attendance, this resident did not obtain the competence in terms of the number of attempts (red line).

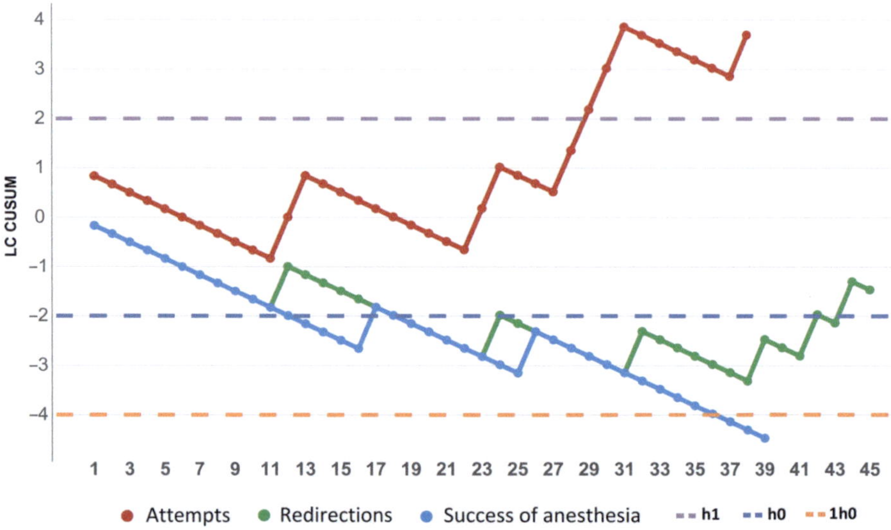


**Fig. 10** The LC CUSUM curve showing the resident not getting the competence: number of attempts skill (red line)

We believe that those responsible for training should establish a clear method for determining what is an acceptable failure rate for the administration of the epidural block and other practical procedures in anesthesia. So far, this data has been established from the literature, but it could be considered to decide the failure rate based on the actual failure rate of the expert who is about to teach a specific technique.

Kestin [7] retrospectively studied novice trainees (with no previous experience in epidural blocks) and experienced trainees using 5% and 10% as acceptable and unacceptable failure rates and defining failure as "inability to obtain analgesia or anesthesia for any reason." The number of attempts made before crossing the boundary line of the accepted failure rate ranged from 29 to 185 attempts. Only 4 out of 12 trainees (33%) achieved competence in an unspecified period of time.

Naik et al. [8] defined a successful epidural as "an epidural catheter independently positioned that provided some degree of analgesia, without physical assistance from an experienced anesthetist." The trainees self-assessed their scores during the 6 months of training. Using 10% and 15% as acceptable and unacceptable failure rates, they demonstrated that 10 out of 11 subjects (90%) achieved competence after 57 epidural blocks performed during the training period.

Lew et al. [9] have retrospectively studied trainees with no prior experience in combined spinal-epidural anesthesia. The procedure was considered successful if performed with a number of attempts equal to or less than 2. Competence was achieved by 19 out of 24 trainees (79%) after 40 procedures in more than 1 year of training, starting from an acceptable failure rate of 20%.

Regarding the number of attempts needed to achieve competence, our study [4] produced different results compared to those obtained in previous articles that examined competence in performing epidural block using CUSUM analysis.

Our study compared a group of trainees who received a traditional educational model to another group that had received a structured teaching model as described in Chap. "The Structured and Standardized EESOA Model". Setting an acceptable and unacceptable failure rate at 10% and 30%, respectively, the average minimum number of epidurals performed by trainees before reaching competence was only 17 blocks. The most striking result was that the percentage of trainees reaching the level of competence was significantly higher in the group that had participated in the structured epidural teaching model (67% vs 38%).

## 6 Advantages and Limitations of CUSUM Analysis

CUSUM analysis in the context of anesthesia procedures is used to evaluate a specific competence of an anesthetist over time. This evaluation method has advantages and disadvantages.

Among the advantages are:

- The fact that it provides information that can be used to improve training programs and patient outcomes.
- The ability to promptly detect any performance deterioration over time.
- The ability to provide individualized and long-term feedback.
- Greater sensitivity compared to other short-term monitoring techniques that can only provide a snapshot of the medical staff's ability at a given time.
- It can help identify where problems lie in the medical procedure and/or the anesthetist's performance.

However, there are also some limitations in using the LC-CUSUM curve in monitoring medical procedures:

- The need to standardize the teaching and learning methodology in order to make more accurate comparisons between different clinicians.
- The curve depends on the selection of the parameter chosen to indicate the success of the procedure, which can make it difficult to compare results between different procedures.
- Some of the factors affecting the outcome of the procedure are not under the anesthetist's control, such as physical factors of the patient. In other words, the obstetric epidural block may fail because the parturient is unable to cooperate or due to a defect in drug administration, etc., and these data cannot be included in the CUSUM analysis.
- CUSUM can sometimes be a costly and complicated system to implement, as it requires specific skills for data analysis.

Despite its limitations, if well applied, CUSUM analysis represents a powerful tool for objectively evaluating the performance of medical staff, allowing for timely corrections and/or improvements. However, it is essential to emphasize that it cannot replace a more comprehensive assessment of a professional's clinical abilities.

**Acknowledgments** We thank Dr. Matteo Velardo, statistical consultant, for reviewing this chapter.

## References

1. Wright TP. Factors affecting the cost of airplanes. J Aeronaut Sci. 1936;3:122–8.
2. Hopper AN, Jamison MH, Lewis WG. Learning curves in surgical practice. Postgrad Med J. 2007;83(986):777–9. https://doi.org/10.1136/pgmj.2007.057190.
3. Kopacz DJ, Neal JM, Pollock JE. The regional anesthesia "learning curve". What is the minimum number of epidural and spinal blocks to reach consistency? Reg Anesth. 1996;21:182–90.
4. Scorzoni M, Gonnella GL, Capogna E, Velardo M, Giuri PP, Ciancia M, et al. Achieving lumbar epidural block competency in inexperienced trainees after a structured epidural teaching model: a randomized, single blind, prospective comparison of CUSUM learning curves. Anesthesiol Res Pract. 2022;2022:1738783. https://doi.org/10.1155/2022/1738783.
5. Drake EJ, Coghill J, Sneyd JR. Defining competence in obstetric epidural anaesthesia for inexperienced trainees. BJA. 2015;114:951–571.
6. Sivaprakasam J, Purva M. CUSUM analysis to assess competence: what failure rate is acceptable? Clin Teach. 2010;7:257–61. https://doi.org/10.1111/j.1743-498X.2010.00386.x.
7. Kestin IG. A statistical approach to measuring the competence of anaesthetic trainees at practical procedures. Br J Anaesth. 1995;75:805–9. https://doi.org/10.1093/bja/75.6.805.
8. Naik VN, Devito I, Halpern SH. Cusum analysis is a useful tool to assess resident proficiency at insertion of labour epidurals. Can J Anaesth. 2003;50:694–8. https://doi.org/10.1007/BF03018712.
9. Lew E, Allen JC Jr, Goy RWL, Ithnin F, Sng BL. Determining competence in performing obstetric combined spinal-epidural procedures in junior anesthesiology residents: results from a cumulative sum analysis. Int J Obstet Anesth. 2020;44:33–9. https://doi.org/10.1016/j.ijoa.2020.05.002.

# Teaching with Ultrasounds

Ilaria Pacini

The use of ultrasound before the execution of the neuraxial block promotes the success of the conventional technique, thanks to the accurate identification of the level of the intervertebral space and the midline of the spine and the estimation of the depth of the epidural/subarachnoid space. Although further research is needed to define its role in terms of safety, the most recent scientific evidence reinforces the usefulness of eco-assistance, especially on patient populations with anatomical landmarks difficult to identify, such as obesity, deformities or previous spine surgery.

So far, no methodology has been validated with respect to the teaching of sonoanatomy of the vertebral column. The commonest teaching model is based on conventional modules consisting of a theoretical lesson by an expert; a practical workshop, which usually includes the demonstration on a living model; and a session of practical exercises by the learners.

Nonconventional educational models based on simulation techniques diffused in the last decades. They include cadaver workshops, exercises on a wide variety of mannequin simulators and online lessons on the web. Mannequin simulators, both expensive commercial products and systems manufactured by hand, provide a realistic educational experience and preserve patient safety at the same time. Lastly, technological development has supported the introduction of innovative teaching tools, such as virtual reality.

Currently, there are few data available in the literature regarding the educational effectiveness of conventional, nonconventional and technological models compared to the acquisition of sonoanatomy skills of the spine, so further research is needed to assess the effect of these teaching modules in daily clinical practice, especially on patient populations with expected or unexpected technical difficulties.

I. Pacini (✉)
Department of Anesthesiology, IRCSS Istituto Ortopedico Rizzoli, Bologna, Italy
e-mail: ilariapacini@yahoo.it

© The Author(s), under exclusive license to Springer Nature Switzerland AG 2024

G. Capogna (ed.), *How to Teach the Epidural Block in Obstetric Anesthesia*,
https://doi.org/10.1007/978-3-031-70211-2_5

# 1 Introduction

The use of ultrasound has revolutionized the practice of regional anesthesia in the last two decades, showing considerable advantages over traditional "blind" techniques in terms of time spent in performing procedures and lower incidence of technical failure, resulting in undeniable clinical benefits [1].

However, the clinical use of ultrasound has not consistently affected all areas of regional anesthesia. Contrary to the widespread popularity of application for peripheral regional techniques, the role of ultrasonography before and during the performance of a central block has been underestimated for a long time. This aspect can be primarily attributed to the proven effectiveness, reliability and safety of the traditional technique based on the palpation of anatomical landmarks. Secondly, it may be due to the complexity of technical execution in identifying an acoustic window favorable to the visualization of the target, namely the spinal canal and its content. In fact, the latter represent deep anatomical structures protected by a complex bone structure, the vertebral column, which hinders the passage of ultrasound, except for two points, represented by the interlaminar space and the interspinous space [2] (Fig. 1).

However, the conventional "blind" technique could be complex and traumatic, requiring multiple attempts, or even fail, especially in those pathological conditions that do not allow the accurate identification of anatomical landmarks, such as obesity and spinal deformities (scoliosis, degenerative diseases of the spine, or previous spine surgery). The physiological changes that occur during pregnancy, such as

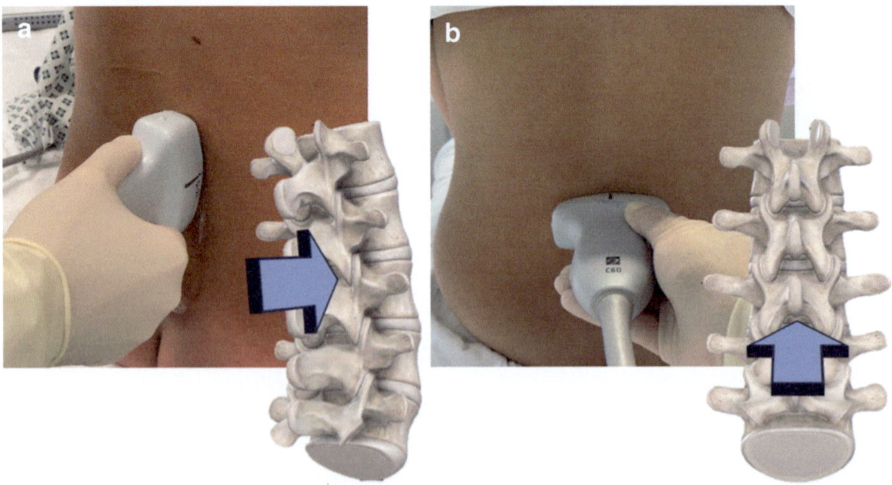


**Fig. 1** (**a**) The ultrasound probe is oriented parallel to the longitudinal axis of the spine, 1–2 cm laterally from the median interspinous line and with a slight angulation in the latero-medial direction in such a way that the ultrasound beam aligns with the interlaminar space. (**b**) The ultrasound probe is oriented perpendicular to the longitudinal axis of the spine, in such a way as to orient the ultrasound beam according to the interspinous space

increased body weight, the presence of soft tissue edema and the accentuation of lumbar lordosis, can also compromise the identification of classic anatomical references. Moreover, other factors can contribute to making the regional technique more challenging in obstetric patients. They are represented by the laxity of the ligaments, which can alter the tactile sensation of loss of resistance during the retrieval of the epidural space, the limitation of the bending of the spine due to the pregnant uterus that can hinder the optimal positioning of the patient, and, finally, the concomitance of the pathological conditions mentioned above [3].

In such contexts, the use of ultrasound before the execution of the neuraxial block allows to obtain additional anatomical information, that is, the accurate identification of the level of the intervertebral space and the midline and the estimation of the depth of the epidural/subarachnoid space, which promote the success of the conventional technique. Although further research is needed to define its role in terms of safety, the most recent scientific evidence reinforces the usefulness of eco-assistance, especially where technical difficulties are expected or are encountered [4].

## 2 Technical Description

Ultrasound scanning of the lumbar spine before the execution of a central block (eco-assistance) involves the use of a low frequency (2–5 MHz), curved array ultrasound probe (convex) which allows the ultrasonic beam to penetrate into the deeper anatomical structures.

Before proceeding with the scan, it is essential to know and change some functions of the ultrasound machine, in order to optimize the image quality on the screen:

1. **Depth**: this parameter should be set in relation to the depth at which the target structure is expected to be found and according to the patient's conformation. Usually, it is selected in a variable range between 6 and 13 cm.
2. **Gain**: represents the function that makes the ultrasound image brighter, through signal amplification. In some ultrasound machines, it is possible to optimize the gain through the time gain compensation (earnings slide), which affects individual areas of the screen located at different depths. Alternatively, the total gain, which strengthens the signal over the entire field.
3. **Focus**: is the tool that allows the ultrasound beam to converge at a certain depth, improving the resolution of the image. It is positioned at the depth of the target structure.
4. The selection of the lowest frequency in the convex probe range.

The probe is oriented according to the paramedian sagittal oblique plane and the median transverse plane, with the patient in a sitting (Fig. 2) or lateral decubitus position (Fig. 3). In the absence of contraindications, it is also possible to perform the scan with the patient in the prone position. Through these two planes of

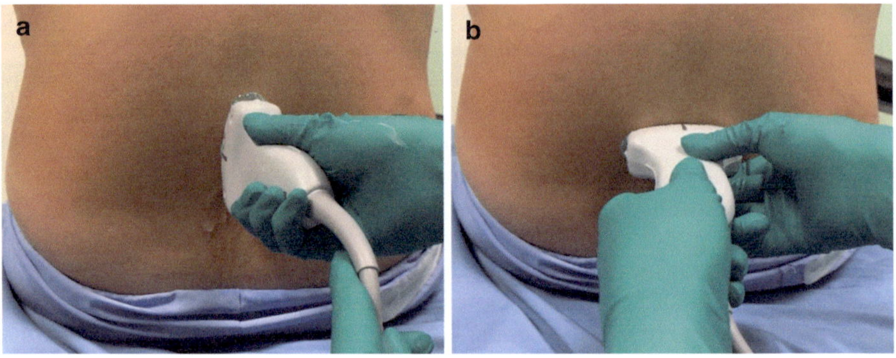


**Fig. 2** (**a**) Probe oriented according to the paramedian sagittal oblique plane with the patient in a sitting position. (**b**) Probe oriented according to the median transverse plane with the patient in a sitting position

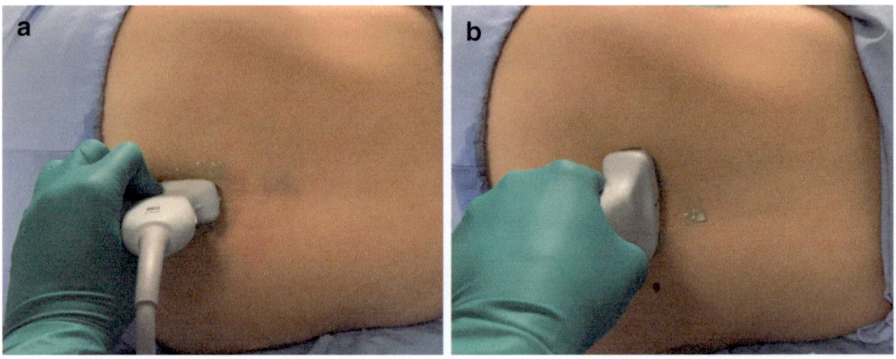


**Fig. 3** (**a**) Probe oriented according to the paramedian sagittal oblique plane with the patient in a lateral decubitus position. (**b**) Probe oriented according to the median transverse plane with the patient in a lateral decubitus position

ultrasound scanning, it is possible to obtain the following useful information before proceeding with the neuraxial block:

- Accurate identification of the level of a specific lumbar interspace.
- Localization of the median point of the lumbar spine.
- Accurate estimation of the depth of the epidural/intrathecal space, that is, the depth of insertion of the spinal needle or Tuohy needle.
- Prediction of the needle's inclination based on the cranio-caudal tilting of the probe [5].

***Oblique Paramedian Sagittal Scan*** The ultrasound probe is oriented parallel to the longitudinal axis of the spine, 1–2 cm laterally from the median interspinous line, at

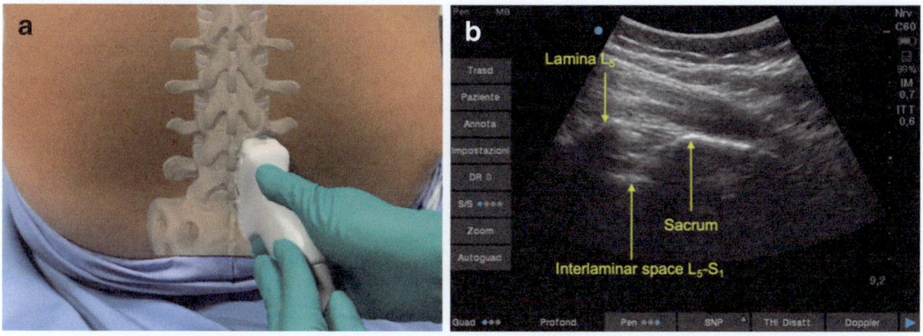


**Fig. 4** (**a**) Paramedian sagittal oblique scan of the lumbar spine at the level of the sacrum and the fifth lumbar vertebra ($L_5$). (**b**) Paramedian sagittal oblique sonogram showing the sacrum, as a flat and hyperechoic line; the lamina of the fifth lumbar vertebra ($L_5$); and the $L_5$-$S_1$ interlaminar space, as a gap between the sacrum and the lamina of the $L_5$ vertebra

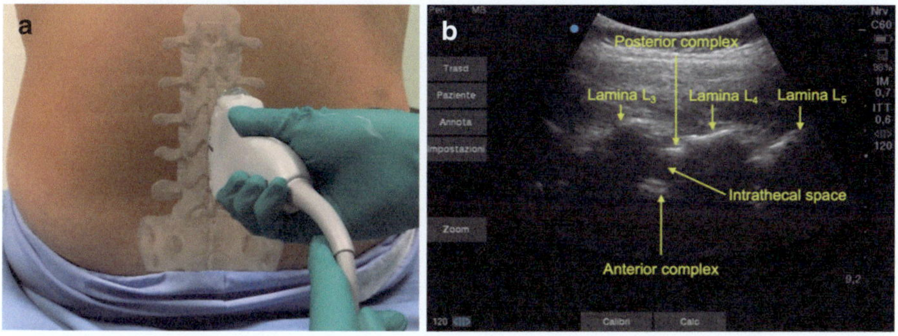


**Fig. 5** (**a**) Paramedian sagittal oblique scan of the lumbar spine at the level of the third ($L_3$), the fourth ($L_4$), and the fifth lumbar vertebra ($L_5$). (**b**) Paramedian sagittal oblique sonogram showing the typical hyperechoic image, defined "sawtooth" (Saw-tooth). Each hyperechoic protrusion (tooth) of this line identifies the lamina of the vertebra, with the respective acoustic shadow anterior to each lamina. The gap between the hyperechoic lines of the laminae represents the paramedian interlaminar space, where the posterior complex and the anterior complex are identified in the posteroanterior direction

the level of the sacral promontory. Subsequently, a slight angulation in the latero-medial direction (latero-medial tilting) allows the ultrasound beam to be oriented towards the vertebral canal and its content (Figs. 4a and 5a). It visualizes, therefore, a continuous hyperechoic line that represents the sacrum (Fig 4b). Advancing the probe in the cephalic direction, the hyperechoic rhyme stops at the interlaminar space of $L_5$-$S_1$ (also defined gap $L_5$-$S_1$) and the typical hyperechoic image, defined "sawtooth" (**saw-tooth**), appears. Each protrusion (tooth) of this line identifies the lamina of the vertebra, with the respective acoustic shadow. The interruption (gap) between the hyperechoic lines of the laminae represents the paramedian interlaminar space. At the level of each interlaminar space, it is possible to identify the following structures in the posteroanterior direction:

- **The posterior complex**: consisting of the ligamentum flavum, the epidural space and the posterior portion of the dura. The set of these structures usually appears as a single hyperechoic rhyme. In some cases, it is possible to distinguish the ligamentum flavum as a more superficial hyperechoic rhyme, separated by a hypoechoic space (the epidural space) from the deeper hyperechoic line, which identifies the posterior dura.
- **The intrathecal space** (hypo-anechoic).
- **The anterior complex**: consisting of the anterior part of the dura, the posterior longitudinal ligament and the vertebral body, visible as a single hyperechoic line (Fig 5b).

The movement of the ultrasound probe in the cranial direction, starting from the sacrum and the interlaminar space $L_5$-$S_1$, allows the level of the intervertebral spaces to be accurately determined by using the laminae as a reference (**counting-up**). Finally, at a specific interspace, it is possible to measure the depth of the ligamentum flavum-epidural space with respect to the parasagittal plane, using the calibration software [5].

The scientific evidence available so far has shown that ultrasonography of the spine allows the intervertebral spaces to be identified with greater accuracy compared to palpable anatomical landmarks on the skin surface (grade B recommendation) [6].

***Transverse Scanning at the Midline Level*** At the interspace identified through the paramedian longitudinal scan, the ultrasound probe is rotated 90°, perpendicular to the longitudinal axis of the spine, in such a way as to orient the ultrasound beam according to the transverse plane (Figs. 6a, 7a and 8a). If the ultrasound beam cor-

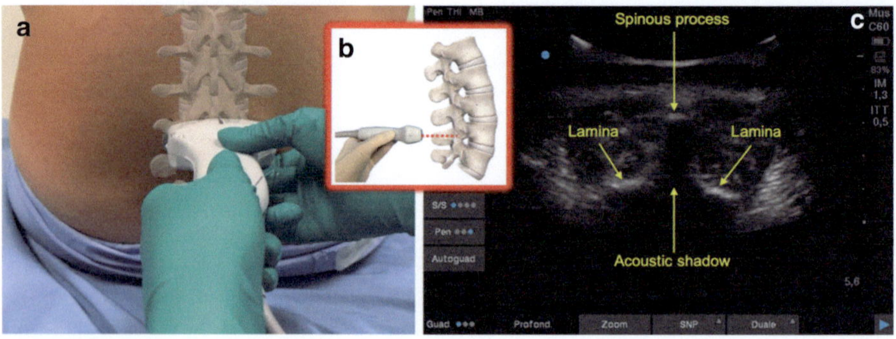


**Fig. 6** (**a**) Transverse scan of the lumbar spine with the transducer oriented perpendicular to the longitudinal axis of the spine and (**b**) the ultrasound beam corresponding to the $L_4$ spinous process. (**c**) Transverse sonogram showing the tip of spinous process, as a small hyperechoic rhyme, immediately below the skin plane, with a deeper acoustic shadow or a hypoechoic triangular image, which occupies most of the screen, obscuring the spinal canal and the neuraxial structures. The sides of the triangular area are delimited by two hyperechoic rhymes, which correspond to the laminae

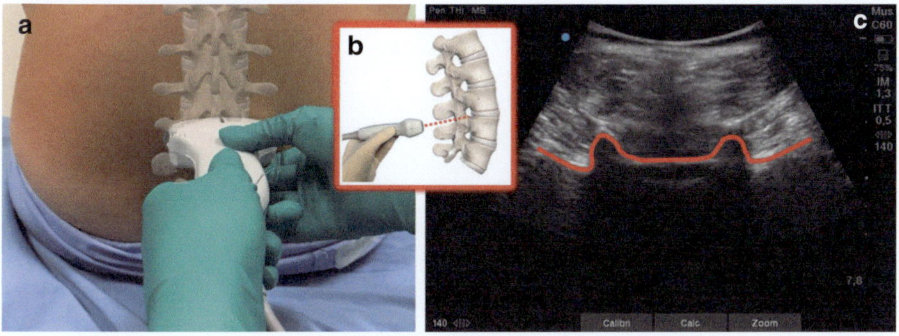


**Fig. 7** (**a**) Transverse scan of the lumbar spine with the transducer oriented perpendicular to the longitudinal axis of the spine and (**b**) the ultrasound beam aligning with the interspinous/interlaminar space between the third ($L_3$) and the fourth ($L_4$) vertebra. (**c**) Transverse sonogram showing the typical reference model, called "bat wings" (Flying bat) image (red line)

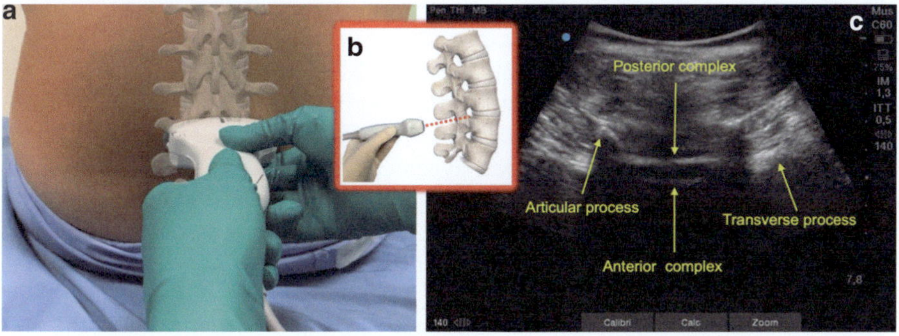


**Fig. 8** (**a**) Transverse scan of the lumbar spine with the transducer oriented perpendicular to the longitudinal axis of the spine and (**b**) the ultrasound beam aligning with the interspinous/interlaminar space between the third ($L_3$) and the fourth ($L_4$) vertebra. (**c**) Transverse sonogram showing the posterior complex, as the most superficial hyperechoic rhyme, consisting of the ligamentum flavum, the epidural space, and the posterior portion of the dura; the intrathecal space (hypoanechoic); the anterior complex, as the deepest hyperechoic line; the lateral paramedian structures: the articular processes (more superficial) and transverse processes (deeper)

responds to the spinous process (Fig 6b), the tip of the latter will be displayed as a small hyperechoic rhyme, immediately below the skin plane, with a deeper acoustic shadow or a hypoechoic triangular image, which occupies most of the screen. The sides of this triangular area are delimited by two hyperechoic rhymes, which correspond to the laminae (Fig 6c).

Sliding the probe in the cranial or caudal direction, simultaneously with a slight inclination (cranial or caudal tilting), allows the bone obstacle represented by the spinous process to be overcome, in such a way that the ultrasound beam aligns with the interspinous/interlaminar space so permitting the view of the vertebral canal and

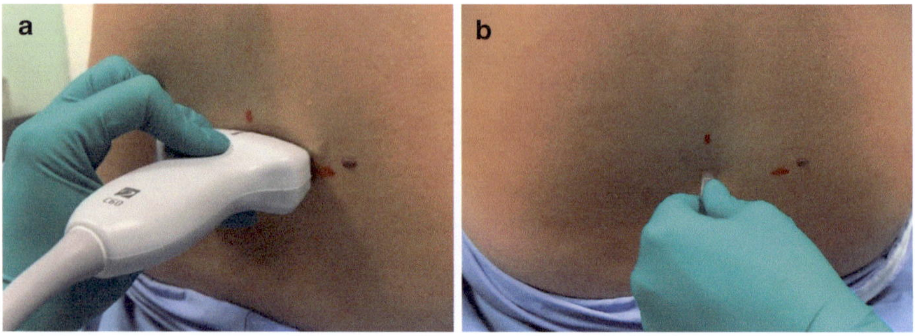


**Fig. 9** (**a**) Marking on the skin the midpoint of the long axis and the midpoint of the short axis of the probe. (**b**) The insertion point of the epidural/spinal needle is obtained from the intersection of the two points

its content (Figs. 7b and 8b). The sonographic reference model is called "bat wings" (**Flying bat**) image (Fig 7c) and identifies the following anatomical structures:

- **The posterior complex**: the most superficial hyperechoic rhyme, consisting of the ligamentum flavum, the epidural space and the posterior portion of the dura.
- **The intrathecal space** (hypo-anechoic).
- **The anterior complex**: the deepest hyperechoic line, consisting of the anterior part of the dura, the posterior longitudinal ligament and the vertebral body.
- **The lateral paramedian structures**, i.e. the articular processes (more superficial) and transverse processes (deeper) (Fig. 8c).

Once the echographic landmarks are identified, the insertion point of the epidural/spinal needle is obtained from the intersection between the midpoint of the long axis and the midpoint of the short axis of the probe (Fig. 9). Moreover, through this approach, it is possible, by using the calibration software, to measure the distance between the skin plane and the deepest limit of the posterior complex on the midline and accurately estimate the depth of the epidural/intrathecal space [5] (Fig. 10).

In this regard, the literature has shown that spinal ultrasound can be used to accurately predict the depth of needle insertion to reach the epidural space or intrathecal space (grade A recommendation). There is a close correlation between the two measures, i.e. the estimate of the distance of the skin-epidural space measured on the ultrasound image and the actual depth of insertion of the needle. Nevertheless, such measures may not always coincide. It has been estimated that the difference between the two measures could vary in the range between 1 and 13 mm. Ultrasound measurement usually tends to underestimate the actual depth of needle insertion, mainly due to surface tissue compression exerted by the ultrasound probe [6].

Finally, the trajectory traversed by the needle during insertion reflects the angle of the ultrasound probe on the transverse plane that allowed the optimal insonation of the target (flying-bat ultrasound image) [5].

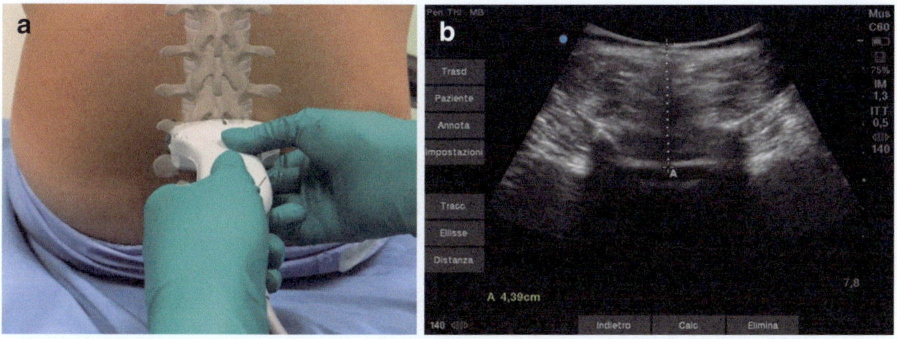


**Fig. 10** (**a**) Transverse scan of the lumbar spine with the transducer oriented perpendicular to the longitudinal axis of the spine and the ultrasound beam aligning with the interspinous/interlaminar space. (**b**) The distance between the skin plane and the deepest limit of the posterior complex on the midline, by using the calibration software

## 3 The Conventional Teaching Model

The awareness of the advantages deriving from ultrasound assistance before performing a neuraxial block has favored in recent years a considerable interest also in the didactic and training aspects related to the sonoanatomy of the spine, which, like the complexity of technical execution, are particularly difficult to understand [7].

So far, no methodology has been validated with respect to the teaching of this discipline. The proposed models are quite similar to each other and over the years have been gradually enriched with innovative teaching modules, also thanks to the concomitant technological progress. Only for some of them, the effectiveness of training aimed at the recognition of the anatomical structures of the spine has been evaluated [8]. However, further investigation is needed to assess the effect of these teaching modules in daily clinical practice, especially on patient populations with anatomical landmarks difficult to identify or with expected or unexpected technical difficulties.

The training path for the acquisition of the necessary skills to perform an ultrasound scan of the spine is divided into two phases:

1. The first phase, purely theoretical, consists in achieving the skills necessary to recognize the eco-anatomical structures on the screen and to be able to interpret them in the clinical context.
2. The second is represented by the acquisition of conventional manual skills that allow practitioners to:
   (a) Be able to manipulate and orient the ultrasound probe in order to acquire an acoustic window favorable to the identification of target anatomical structures.
   (b) Be able to identify the level of a certain intervertebral space and the median point of the spine on the patient's skin, in order to determine the exact point of needle insertion.

(c) Be able to measure and estimate the depth of the epidural/subarachnoid space [9].

The training course cannot be separated from the knowledge of the basics of anatomy and sonoanatomy of the spine. Therefore, it presupposes individual study, preferably preceded by a theoretical lesson by an expert, who, in our opinion, does not simply have the role of making the explanation of the notions simpler and more accessible, but also to make learners aware of the usefulness of the eco-assisted procedure, against which, often, they show great distrust. Echo-assisted central blocks represent advanced regional anesthesia procedures and require the acquisition of the abovementioned skills with experience and practice. For this reason, the next phase always involves a practical workshop, which usually includes the demonstration on a living model by an expert tutor and, subsequently, a session of practical exercises by the learners. It is preferable that the practical workshop is carried out, at least at the initial phase, on healthy living models with physiological anatomy. The limitation of the practical part is that, although it allows the ultrasound probe to be manipulated in the exercise, in order to acquire the correct acoustic window and to identify the reference anatomical structures on the ultrasound image, it cannot verify that the needle insertion point is actually correct, nor does it highlight the correspondence between the depth of the posterior complex estimated on the ultrasound image and the actual depth of needle insertion or to estimate the inclination of the needle with respect to the orientation of the probe. For this reason, it is useful for the theoretical lesson to be accompanied by explanatory videos of the entire procedure, including the performance of the anesthetic technique and the variants of the physiological sonoanatomy found in the most frequently encountered pathological conditions in clinical practice, such as obesity and scoliosis. There is no unanimity in the literature even with respect to the definition of "expert in the sonoanatomy of the spine," although in most cases, it refers to a specialist in anesthesia and resuscitation with at least 4 years of clinical experience of vertebral sonoanatomy.

Finally, the training course should conclude with the practice on patients under the supervision of the tutor. Obviously this last one, despite its undeniable educational value, is subject to significant ethical restrictions, as it is essential to always ensure the safety and the comfort of the patient during each maneuver and to respect the timing of its use. Consider, for example, possible delays in the administration of labor analgesia in a pregnant patient or the difficulty for the patient to maintain the position for a long time, first during ultrasound procedures and then during the execution of the anesthetic technique.

The literature reports that the development of the skills necessary to correctly perform an ultrasound scan of the spine is far from simple. In 2010, Margarido C. B. et al. published a study on the learning curves of a group of students without any experience in spinal sonoanatomy and subjected to a theoretical and practical educational program. After 7–14 days from theoretical training and practice on healthy living models, the authors showed that none of the 18 participants had acquired the ability to mark the correct injection site on the skin and to estimate the depth of the ligamentum flavum, while only a minority of them (27%) had been able to correctly identify the level of a given intervertebral space, requiring an average number of 11 attempts [7].

The difficulty encountered most frequently by students during the training course was the correct identification of the $L_5$-$S_1$ interspace, while the most common error was inadvertently sliding the probe at least one level caudally during the rotation of the probe from the paramedian sagittal plane to the transverse plane. The study therefore emphasized the need for a more intense practical training session for students, clearly lacking in the proposed educational program, both qualitatively and quantitatively [7].

In a subsequent study, Deacon et al. reported an improvement in the acquisition of sonoanatomical skills by learners, thanks to the adoption of a standardized educational program, based on the adoption of a protocol consisting of ten simple steps for the execution of the procedure and a more intensive individual practical session [10]. In order to construct the learning curves, the sequence of attempts performed by the participants was elaborated through the cumulative sum analysis model (CUSUM) (reference to Chap. "Learning Curves"). It was found that all learners were able to correctly identify a given interlaminar space after an average number of 5 attempts and to accurately measure the depth of the posterior complex after about 40 attempts (average number of 10). However, as shown in Margarido et al.'s study, the correct identification of the needle insertion point was a difficult skill to learn. Only two out of the five participants showed the acquisition of this ability after 55 ultrasound scans, considering 5 mm as the maximum error limit compared to the expert measure. On the other hand, by tolerating an upper error limit (8 mm), all learners were able to correctly mark the needle insertion point on the skin, showing that the success rate in achieving a given competence on the part of the learner depends not only on the intrinsic complexity of the competence but also on the accuracy of the student and the accuracy imposed by the examiner [10].

The results of other authors have highlighted the need to perform a minimum of 20 ultrasound scans in order to reach the minimum threshold of skills for the sonoanatomy of the spine [4]. This data was further supported by a study conducted in patients between the ages of 3 and 20 years about to undergo urgent lumbar puncture. The authors concluded that 19 attempts were insufficient to achieve the necessary skills to carry out the eco-assisted procedure [11]. The peculiarity of this study is that, unlike the previous ones, performed on healthy models, it was carried out on patients who accessed the facility for diagnostic lumbar puncture and that the participants' technical skills were evaluated over a long period of time, specifically 3 months. In addition to reaffirming the concept of the quantitative importance of practical exercises, this study highlighted the need for continuous training for the learner, extended over a long period of time, and on patients with different anatomical characteristics. In this regard, the work of Terblanche et al. showed that repetitive training, with guidance and feedback from an expert, favored the acquisition of skills by the learner, representing a fundamental and essential element of the teaching program of vertebral eco-assistance [12].

## 4 Nonconventional and Innovative Educational Models

The focus on patient safety has contributed to increasing interest in simulation techniques in regional anesthesia training. The intent to provide a realistic educational experience in order to preserve patient safety has consolidated over the years [13]. Today, simulation-based teaching is an essential component of peripheral regional anesthesia teaching programs and, albeit more contained, of ultrasound-assisted and ultrasound-guided spinal procedures. This interest, however, is destined to grow due to the spread and popularity of pain therapy techniques that involve this anatomical district. The simulation models are multiple and include cadaver workshops, exercises on a wide variety of mannequin simulators with courses carried out in specific centers and online lessons on the web. Moreover, technological development has supported the introduction of innovative teaching tools, such as virtual reality. However, it is necessary to underline that currently there are few data available in the literature regarding the educational effectiveness of these technological tools compared to the acquisition of sonoanatomy skills of the spine.

### 4.1 Cadaver Workshop

The exercise on fresh cadavers or alternatively subjected to preservation procedures (for example, the Thiel embalming technique) [14] allows students to accurately study the sonoanatomy of the spine and practice echo-assisted/echo-guided procedures, providing realistic tactile feedback [15]. However, the limitations are represented that these models sometimes offer poor-quality ultrasound images and the limited availability of corpses that can be used for educational purposes. For these reasons, the available courses are quite rare and very expensive and it is possible to participate only in selected anatomy institutes.

### 4.2 Workshops on Animals

Pigs subjected to general anesthesia are very useful models for teaching and practicing spinal ultrasound, which closely resembles human anatomy. Moreover, they represent a very useful and reliable tool for performing echo-guided techniques. However, to carry out such courses, it is necessary to obtain the approval from the animal ethics committee and special authorizations. Moreover, ethical and religious limitations and potential infectious risks limit their diffusion [16].

### 4.3 Mannequin Simulators

There are several varieties of mannequin simulators that can be used not only for the execution of spinal and epidural anesthesia but also for the eco-assistance of the spine and the central echo-guided block. They include both particularly sophisticated and expensive commercial products and systems manufactured by hand and economically more sustainable, but equally useful.

The simplest model for the study of the sonoanatomy of the lumbar spine, called "water-based phantom thorns," consisted of a model of a lumbosacral column immersed in a basin containing water, in such a way as to cover the extremities of the spiny processes facing 1–2 cm above. The ultrasound scans were performed according to the sagittal and transverse plane, with the ultrasound probe in contact with the water (Fig. 11) [17]. It was a very economical tool, easy and quick to reproduce and very useful from an educational point of view, allowing the easy identification of the reflecting, hyperechoic-looking bone surfaces surrounded by anecogen water [18]. However, it was replaced by more complex models, also able to reproduce the soft tissues surrounding the bone structures.

The description of one of the first successful handmade models dates back to 2011 [16]. It is a mannequin simulator in which a model of the lumbosacral column was immersed in a compound consisting of gelatin, agar and water, appropriately mixed and subjected to a subsequent solidification process, able to mimic ultrasound soft tissues surrounding the spine (Fig. 12) [17]. During ultrasound scans, the

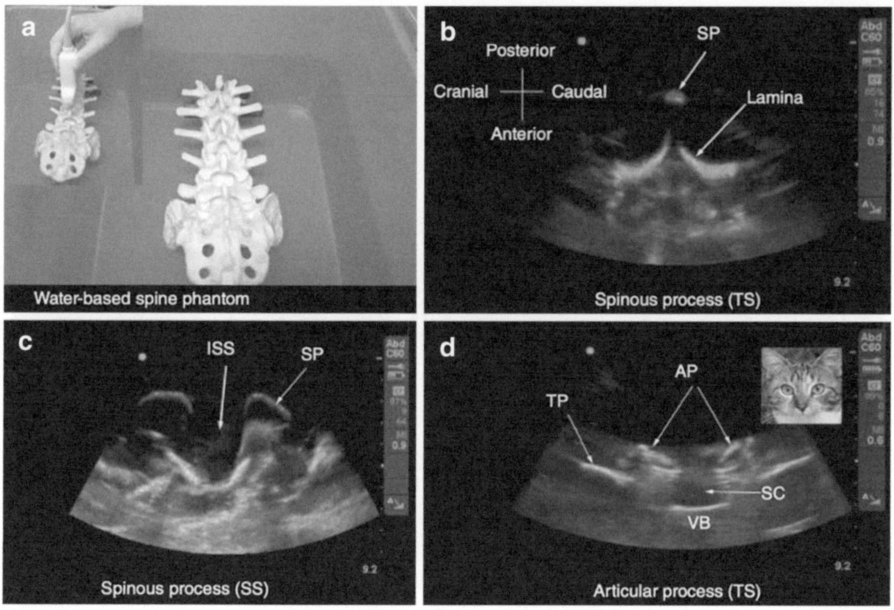


**Fig. 11** (**a**) The water-based spine phantom. The lumbosacral spine is immersed in a water bath and imaged through the water using a curved linear transducer. The other images are sonograms from the water-based lumbosacral spine phantom showing (**b**) the transverse spinous process (SP) view, (**c**) the median sagittal spinous process view, and (**d**) the transverse interspinous view. An inset image has been placed next to **d** to illustrate the resemblance of the sonographic appearance of the transverse interspinous view to a cat's head; hence, this is referred to as the "cat's head sign." *AP* articular process, *ISS* interspinous space, *SC* spinal canal, *SP* spinous process, *SS* sagittal scan, *TP* transverse process, *TS* transverse scan, *VB* vertebral body. From [17] with permission

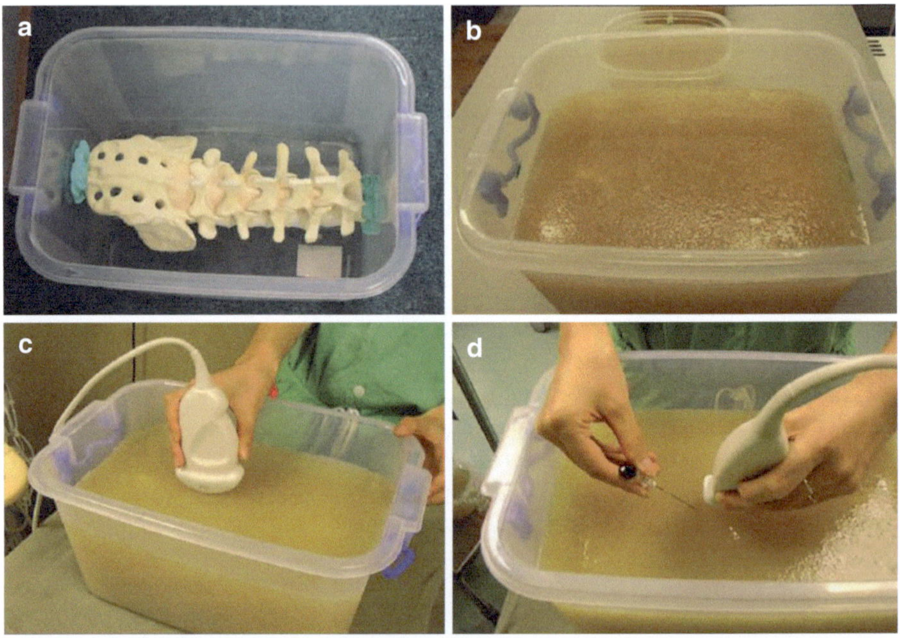


**Fig. 12** Gelatin–agar spine phantom. (**a**) Lumbosacral spine model secured to the base of the plastic box. (**b**) Spine phantom after being embedded in the gelatin–agar mixture. (**c**) Performing a US scan of the gelatin–agar spine phantom. (**d**) Simulated in-plane needle insertion in the gelatin–agar spine phantom. From [17] with permission

model has been shown to reproduce quite faithfully the spine of the living, proving to be a valuable tool for teaching the sonoanatomy of the spine, for the exercise of echo-guided procedures and having leading advantages compared to previous models (Fig. 13). Compared to models made only with gelatin, in fact, this new simulator had the advantage of being opaque and, therefore, made impossible the visualization of the bone structure embedded in the compound, allowing the operator to focus only on the image displayed on the ultrasound screen. At the same time, compared to other models, based on the author's experience, it has proven to be more resistant to wear caused by the insertion of needles during the execution of echo-guided procedures. Moreover, the addition of chlorhexidine to the compound has allowed the growth of molds and bacteria on its surface to be delayed and, therefore, has permitted its use for an extended period of up to 4 months and repeated use by about 200 learners. However, the limitation of this model was the lack of reproduction of other tissues, such as ligaments, meninges and cerebrospinal fluid, and, therefore, the lack of tactile feedback during the performance of echo-guided procedures. Since then, other handcrafted models have been proposed through the use of different materials, equally resistant and durable and capable of faithfully reproducing the palpation of anatomical landmarks, while maintaining the ecogenic characteristics. Noteworthy, a 3D lumbosacral spine model has been reproduced through

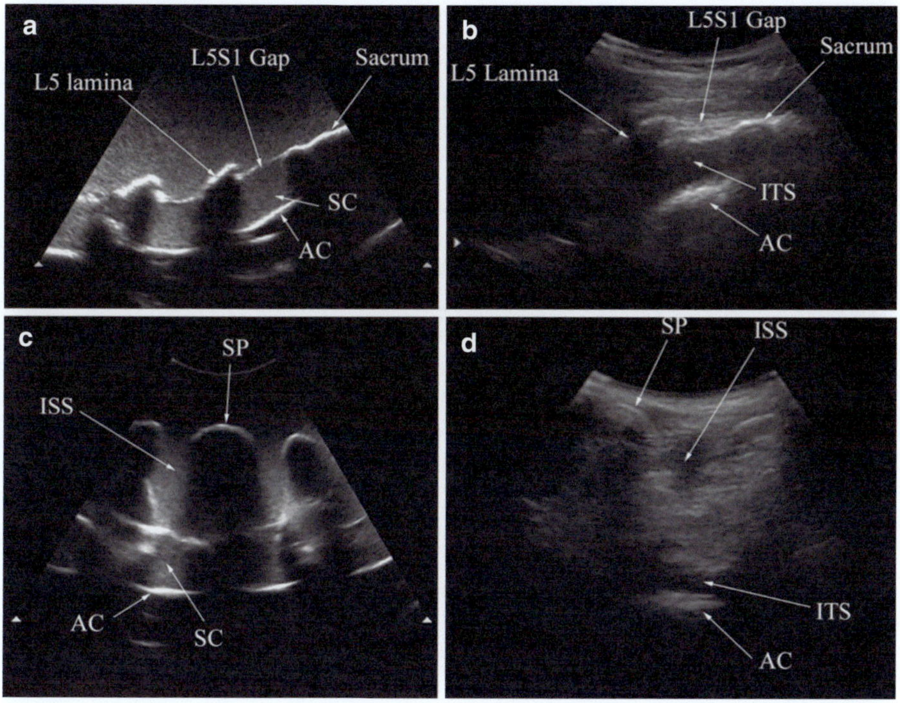


**Fig. 13** Sagittal sonograms of the $L_5$-$S_1$ gap (**a**, **b**) and the spinous processes (**c**, **d**) from the gelatin–agar spine phantom (**a**, **c**) and volunteers (**b**, **d**). *AC* anterior complex, *ISS* interspinous space, *ITS* intrathecal sac, *SC* spinal canal, *SP* spinous processes

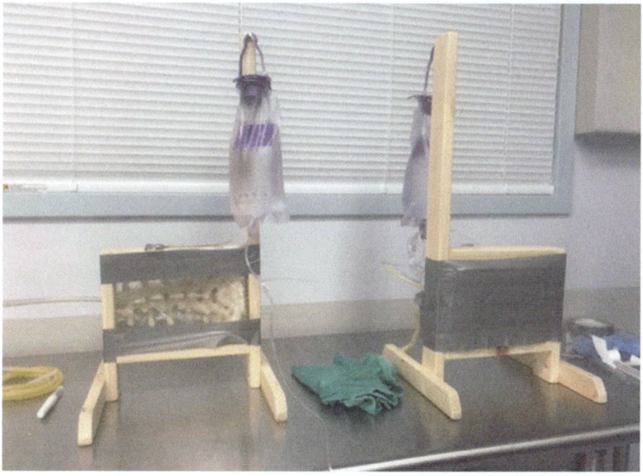

**Fig. 14** Completed lumbar punctures model before and after concealment. Latex tubing inserted within the spine model at the site of spinal canal was connected to a fluid reservoir (500 ml normal saline bag) to simulate the cerebrospinal fluid (CSF) reservoir. From [19] with permission

computerized cadaver tomographic scanning without vertebral pathologies and surrounded by ballistic gelatin, for soft tissue reproduction and with ecogenic properties (Fig. 14) [19].

In the literature, the effectiveness of the use of mannequin simulators for subarachnoid/epidural anesthesia and having ecogenic properties compared to the acquisition of skills of vertebral sonoanatomy is not described. However, the use of simulators made with gelatin enriched with psyllium fibers has been successfully reported in the teaching training of some echo-guided pain therapy procedures, such as the infiltration of articular facets [20].

Unlike handcrafted models, commercial simulators are more expensive, but equipped with features and reproduction fidelity extremely close to the reality of clinical practice. There are several models for the simulation of the central blocks and some of them are ecogenic; that is, they are constructed with materials that simulate the acoustic properties of human tissues (for example, the SimulexUS material of the simulator Blue Phantom$^{R}$) and, therefore, represent a potential teaching tool (ref. to the Chapter on Epidural Simulators).

Technology in relation to mannequin simulators is constantly evolving in the field of regional anesthesia and it is expected that in the near future, more resources will be invested in integrating them into the educational programs of sonoanatomy of the spine, at the moment unfortunately still very limited, possibly also having models with anatomical variants, such as skeletal deformities. Finally, it is necessary to verify how these new teaching and exercise tools act on students' learning curves.

## 4.4 Online Simulation Courses

Currently, videos and simulation courses related to spinal sonoanatomy are available on the web. Noteworthy, a model is divided into three modules: the first concerning vertebral anatomy, the second the sonoanatomy of the lumbar spine and the third a simulation of the exploratory scanning of the spine, equipped with the possibility of virtual manipulation of the ultrasound probe, in order to obtain the acoustic window favorable to the visualization of the reference anatomical structures. This model, properly integrated into conventional teaching programs, has shown to improve students' performance of the correct identification of the levels of intervertebral spaces, of the median and of the point of needle insertion. Despite the limitations of such virtual models, such as the lack of tactile feedback and perception of the need to apply in some cases a certain compression by the ultrasound probe on soft tissues to improve the visualization of anatomical structures, they still reinforce the need for practical exercise and their educational value, even if exclusively for individual deepening, which can be carried out anywhere and without time constraints. It has still to be defined, however, whether such simulation models can play a role in promoting the operator's first attempt success, during the execution of the anesthetic procedure in vivo [21].

### 4.5 Virtual Reality

More recently, technological advances have allowed the introduction of high fidelity fully immersive virtual reality or a completely digital three-dimensional experiential environment, generated by the computer. Unlike traditional user interfaces that only allow users to view a screen, fully immersive virtual reality allows the user to enter an experience, immerse themselves and interact with a three-dimensional world, ensuring a very realistic simulation experience. The use of special gloves equipped with sensors allows movements, the manipulation of objects in the virtual environment and, therefore, can be used to develop certain skills. Currently, the focus in the application of such teaching tools is on the acquisition of motor skills, such as needle guidance during the execution of locoregional procedures. The potential advantages are represented by avoiding the use of commercial simulators, which tend to deteriorate with prolonged use, and biological simulators, which have limited usage time and immediate feedback regarding the performance executed by the software, graphically represented by the custom learning curve. At the moment, there are no data available regarding the use of such teaching tools applied in the teaching of the sonoanatomy of the spine; however, it is worthy of future exploration [22].

## 5 Ultrasound Assistance of the Spine in Cases of Expected or Unexpected Technical Difficulties

At the conclusion of this discussion, it is necessary to emphasize the role of ultrasound in all those clinical situations that represent expected or unexpected technical difficulties. We believe it is a fundamental part of the training process to sensitize students to the role of spinal ultrasound assistance in the most difficult clinical situations, such as severe obesity, to promote the success of neuraxial procedures, highlighting that in many of these circumstances, even if it is not possible to obtain all four points mentioned in the sonoanatomical information above, the use of ultrasound is still decisive in identifying the median of the spine or in demonstrating the presence of a skeletal deformity not clearly perceptible by palpation alone. It is the demonstration of the success of ultrasound in terms of reducing the risk of technical failure and the number of attempts compared to the blind technique that convinces the most skeptical students of the clinical importance of this discipline.

The most recent meta-analyses allow us to affirm that spinal ultrasound improves the effectiveness of epidural and subarachnoid anesthesia, through the reduction of the risk of technical failure and the number of necessary attempts, both in patients with palpable anatomical landmarks and in patients where technical difficulties are expected, such as obesity, scoliosis or previous spine surgery (grade A recommendation) [6]. In particular, it has been estimated that the use of ultrasound reduces the risk of technical failure by 31% compared to the traditional technique. Moreover, considering only the subgroup of patients with expected technical difficulty, the risk reduction increases to 47% [23]. Finally, it has been shown that spinal ultrasound can help improve the safety of neuraxial anesthesia (grade B recommendation) [6].

The following description is illustrative of the use of spinal ultrasound assistance in the obese obstetric patient and the strategies that can be adopted to improve image resolution, which in these patients is not optimal.

Obesity can be associated with difficulty in palpating the spinous processes and the iliac crests and in recognizing the midline and the intervertebral spaces of the spine. Moreover, adipose infiltration increases the incidence of false positives during attempts to locate the epidural space, the event of accidental puncture of the dura mater and vascular puncture and failure of the neuraxial technique is more frequent [24].

On the other hand, with current sonographic techniques, image resolution is not optimal in the obese patient, as the target structure (posterior complex) is located deeper and the ultrasound beam is attenuated by the heterogeneity of the adipose tissue. The presence of artifacts is also very common, as a consequence of the reflection of echoes at the interface between adipose tissue and muscle tissue. This results in a higher percentage of "atypical" ultrasound images on the transverse plane, in which the posterior complex is not identifiable, or even non-resolvable, where no target structure is visible. However, some technical strategies allow us to improve the quality of the ultrasound image and to obtain useful information before proceeding with the puncture:

1. Probe frequency reduction: 2 MHz.
2. Depth adjustment: greater than 9–10 cm.
3. Focus adjustment at the depth level of the transverse process.
4. Compression of the ultrasound probe: by exerting greater compression with the ultrasound probe on the skin plane and the underlying soft tissues, it is possible to improve the sharpness of the ultrasound image, with the intent of bringing the ultrasound beam closer to the target (posterior complex), which in obese patients is located deeper. However, in this way, it is important to be aware that the depth of the epidural space is underestimated.
5. Scanning on the oblique parasagittal plane: very often, the ultrasound image obtained through scanning on the transverse plane does not allow for the identification of the posterior complex and, therefore, the estimation of its depth. However, the images obtained according to this scanning plane are not entirely non-resolutive, because in almost all cases, it is possible to identify the spinous process with the typical deeper acoustic shadow and, therefore, precisely locate the median of the spine, especially in cases where palpation does not allow it. In these cases, scanning on the paramedian sagittal plane offers images of better quality compared to the transverse plane, because avoiding the spinous process allows the use of a window acoustic more favorable to the insonation of the interlaminar space. In this way, the posterior complex is identifiable and it is possible to calculate its depth, because although not identical, it is considered a reliable estimate compared to that obtained on the transverse plane [25] (Fig. 15).

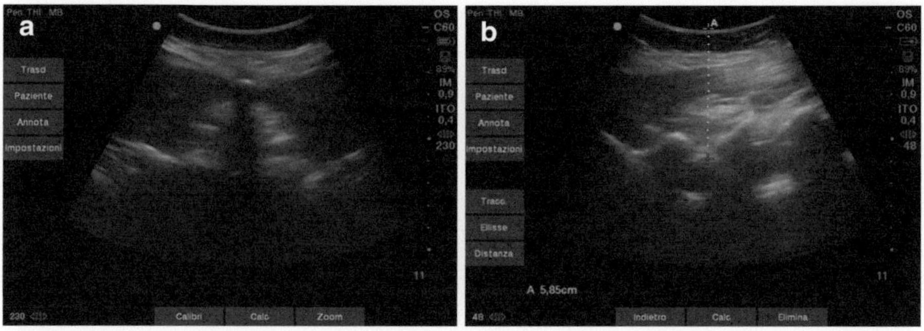


**Fig. 15** (**a**) The ultrasound image obtained through scanning on the transverse plane does not allow for the identification of the posterior complex. (**b**) The posterior complex is identifiable on the paramedian sagittal plane and it is possible to calculate its depth, because it is considered a reliable estimate compared to that obtained on the transverse plane

Contrary to the undeniable advantages, the literature has shown that the clinical use of ultrasound before performing a central block is still very limited. For example, in the United Kingdom, a survey sent to obstetric centers showed that in 2016, the availability of a dedicated ultrasound machine for anesthesiological use was 50.7% and its use mainly concerned the execution of the transversus abdominis plane (TAP) block (56%) and the finding of vascular accesses (52%). Only in 22% of cases was the use intended for the execution of the echo-assisted central block in obstetric patients [26].

Similarly, personal experience, albeit limited, has confirmed the limited spread of echo-assistance of the spinal column among the skills of specialist anesthesiologist colleagues and those in specialist training. We are aware that over the course of these years, the confidence of the learners towards ultrasound has increased, thanks to the spread of its use in other areas of anesthesiology and resuscitation and therefore, it would be interesting to propose studies on learning curves today, to see if the evolution of recent years can positively influence the learning of students. We believe it is appropriate, therefore, that greater attention should be paid to the teaching of this discipline, starting from the introduction of its teaching in specialist training programs and in the search for innovative and effective teaching tools.

## References

1. Albrecht E, Chin KJ. Advances in regional anaesthesia and acute pain management: a narrative review. Anaesthesia. 2020;75(Suppl.1):e101–10.
2. Chin KJ, Karmakar MK, Peng P. Ultrasonography of the adult thoracic and lumbar spine for central neuraxial blockade. Anesthesiology. 2011;114:1459–85.
3. Sadeghi A, Patel R, Carvalho JCA. Ultrasound-facilitated neuraxial anaesthesia in obstetrics. BJA Educ. 21(10):369–75.
4. Balki M, et al. Locating the epidural space in obstetric patients- ultrasound a useful tool: continuing professional development. Can J Anaesth. 2010;57:1111–26.

5. Karmakar MK, Ngan Kee WD, et al. Sonoanatomy relevant for ultrasound-guided central neuraxial blocks via the paramedian approach in the lumbar region. Br J Radiol. 2012;85(1015):e262–e9.
6. Anahi P, Chaparro LE, Chin KJ. Lumbar neuraxial ultrasound for spinal and epidural anesthesia: a systematic review and meta-analysis. Reg Anesth Pain Med. 2016;41(2):251–60.
7. Margarido CB, Arzola C, Balki M, Carvalho JC. Anesthesiologists' learning curves for ultrasound assessment of the lumbar spine. Can J Anaesth. 2010;57:120–6.
8. Vallejo MC, Phelps AL, Singh S, Orebaugh SL, Sah N. Ultrasound decreases the failed labor epidural rate in resident trainees. Int J Obstet Anesth. 2010;19:373–8.
9. Niazi AU, Tait G, Carvalho JC, Chan VW. The use of an online three-dimensional model improves performance in ultrasound scanning of the spine: a randomized trial. Can J Anaesth. 2013;60:458–64.
10. Deacon AJ, Melhuish NS, Terblanche NCS. Cusum method for construction of trainee spinal ultrasound learning curves following standardised teaching. Anaesth Intensive Care. 2014;42:479–85.
11. Rankin JH, Rangarajan V, Chilstrom M, Mailhot T. Learning curves for ultrasound assessment of lumbar puncture insertion sites: when is competency established? J Emerg Med. 2016;51(1):55–62.
12. Terblanche NCS, Arzola C, Wills KE, Lawson R, Blackford D, Balki M. Standardised training program in spinal ultrasound for epidural insertion: protocol-driven versus non–protocol driven teaching approach. Anaesth Intensive Care. 2014;42:459–65.
13. Niazi AU, Haldipur N, Prasad AG, Chan VW. Ultrasound-guided regional anesthesia performance in the early learning period: effect of simulation training. Reg Anesth Pain Med. 2012;37(1):51–4.
14. Ottone NE, Vargas CA, Fuentes R, del Sol M. Walter Thiel's embalming method: review of solutions and applications in different fields of biomedical research. Int J Morphol. 2016;34(4):1442–54.
15. Kessler J, Moriggl B, Grau T. The use of ultrasound improves the accuracy of epidural needle placement in cadavers. Surg Radiol Anat. 2014;36(7):695–703.
16. Li JW, Karmakar MK, Li X, Kwok WH, Ngan Kee WD. Gelatin-agar lumbosacral spine phantom: a simple model for learning the basic skills required to perform real-time sonographically guided central neuraxial blocks. J Ultrasound Med. 2011;30(2):263–72.
17. Admir H, The New York School of Regional Anesthesia Hadzic's textbook of regional anaesthesia and acute pain Management, Second edition 2017, Mc Graw Hill Education. Chapter 40: Karmakar MK and Chin KJ, "Spinal Sonography and Applications of Ultrasound for Central Neuraxial Blocks".
18. Karmakar KM. The "water-based spine phantom"?—a small step towards learning the basics of spinal sonography. BJA. 2009;(103) Issue eLetters Supplement
19. Odom M, Gomez JR, Danelson KA, Sarwal A. Development of a homemade spinal model for simulation to teach ultrasound guidance for lumbar puncture. Neurocrit Care. 2019;31(3):550–8.
20. Kwon ST, et al. The efficacy of lumbosacral spine phantom to improve resident proficiency in performing ultrasound-guided spinal procedure. Pain Med. 2015;16:2284–91.
21. Ramlogan R, Niazi AU, Jin R, Perlas A, et al. A virtual reality simulation model of spinal ultrasound: role in teaching spinal sonoanatomy. Reg Anesth Pain Med. 2017;42(2):217–22.
22. Chuan A, Qian J, Bogdanovych A, Kumar A, McKendrick M, McLeod G. Design and validation of a virtual reality trainer for ultrasound-guided regional anaesthesia. Anaesthesia. 2023;78:739–46.
23. Sidiropoulou T, Christodoulaki K, Siristatidis C. Pre-procedural lumbar neuraxial ultrasound-a systematic review of randomized controlled trials and meta-analysis. Healthcare. 2021;9(4):479.
24. Balki M, Lee Y, Halpern S, Carvalho JC. Ultrasound imaging of the lumbar spine in the transverse plane: the correlation between estimated and actual depth to the epidural space in obese parturients. Anesth Analg. 2009;108(6):1876–81.

25. Singh S, Wirth KM, Phelps AL, Badve MH, Shah TH, Sah N, Vallejo MC. Epidural catheter placement in morbidly obese parturients with the use of an epidural depth equation prior to ultrasound visualization. Sci World J. 2013;2013:695209.
26. Bathia K, et al. The availability and use of ultrasound in UK obstetric anaesthesia. Int J Obstet Anesth. 2016;25:91–2.

# The Structured and Standardized EESOA Model

Giorgio Capogna

The standardized, structured method presented in this chapter is the result of the author's 25 years of practical experience of teaching.

More recently, it has been modified with the addition of the simulator, the construction of the epidural model, and the introduction of new methodologies such as CompuFlo and the EMME method.

This updated educational model is taught at the European School of Obstetric Anesthesia (EESOA) in Rome.

## 1 Module 1: Anatomy—From Bidimensional Vision to 3D Vision for Haptic Perception

*The real voyage of discovery is not to see new worlds, but to change eyes. (Proust)*

The main problems that the teacher faces when teaching epidural anatomy to young doctors in training are due to the widespread assumption that anatomy is already known, that a general knowledge is sufficient for the execution of the technique, and that it is particularly boring. On the other hand, anatomical knowledge of the lumbar epidural region is usually generic or limited to reminiscences of vertebral anatomy with the addition of some schematic notions given by a tutor on the occasion of a previously seen or performed neuraxial block (more often a spinal anesthesia).

G. Capogna (✉)
EESOA European School of Obstetric Anesthesia, Rome, Italy
e-mail: capogna.eesoa@gmail.com

© The Author(s), under exclusive license to Springer Nature Switzerland AG 2024

G. Capogna (ed.), *How to Teach the Epidural Block in Obstetric Anesthesia*,
https://doi.org/10.1007/978-3-031-70211-2_6

## 1.1 Personal Analysis of the Known

The first small step to take is therefore to make students aware of their learning needs.

Each student is given paper and pen, reassuring them that what they write will not be read by the teacher or anyone else, and they are advised not to communicate with each other.

Students are then invited to list on the paper, in 1 min, "the tissues that the needle must pass through to reach the epidural space."

Immediately afterwards, students are asked to write "the tissues that the needle must pass through to reach the epidural space when it is inserted via the paramedian approach."

The question concerning the paramedian approach inevitably raises some doubts, which are exacerbated by the teacher's observation that in clinical practice, the needle is hardly ever inserted perfectly on the midline and that most likely the needle is inserted a few millimeters laterally to what the operator believes to be the "midline."

The most prepared students can correctly identify the ideal path of a needle inserted perfectly on the midline (skin, subcutaneous tissue, supraspinous ligament, interspinous ligament, ligamentum flavum, and epidural space) but generally have strong doubts about which tissues are located a few millimeters laterally from the supraspinous ligament (muscles? which ones? other ligaments? muscle fascia?).

At the end of the test, the teacher does not provide the correct answers, but makes the students imagine that their answers depend on the outcome of the "exam of their life" that will give them access to the best job they can imagine. Immediately afterwards, he asks the students to write on the paper how much anxiety and satisfaction their answers elicited using an analog scale from 0 (none) to 100 (maximum) and then has them turn the paper over and move on to the next session.

This seemingly simple and trivial operational sequence is a powerful means to arouse students' curiosity and to begin to make them aware of their training gaps.

## 1.2 3D Anatomy Laboratory

Even the most prepared students have a two-dimensional view of anatomy, consolidated by the teaching received from teachers who in turn had studied from texts or atlases.

The need for a three-dimensional view is suggested by the teacher who asks the students if they know what haptic sensitivity is. This further step increases the curiosity of the students who learn that, in order to perform a manual "blinded" technique such as an epidural, it is necessary to use their own haptic ability, that is, the sensitivity coming from the combination between the tactile perception of the object on the skin surface (which "reads" its conformation and the more or less smooth or rough nature of the surface) and proprioception, that is, the perception of the position of one's body in relation to the object itself. In this case, the objects that are perceived are the epidural needle, the sensations elicited by the passage of the needle through the tissues, and the spatial position of the needle in relation to the operator. In order to use haptic perception during the execution of an epidural, it is therefore necessary to have a three-dimensional idea not only of the object being used (the needle) but also, and above all, of the tissues being traversed.

And it is for this reason that the transition from a two-dimensional anatomical conception to a three-dimensional one is essential for understanding the anatomical relationships between the tissues that the needle will have to pass through. This transition is achieved by having the students themselves build a three-dimensional model of the lumbar epidural region, which is then consolidated with the aid of slide projections containing traditional anatomical tables, diagrams, and macro- and microphotographs of cadaver sections.

The "surprise effect" of this session is the use of anatomical models with which the students reconstruct the epidural region using easily available materials. The teacher, using the model of the lumbar vertebrae, starting from the explanation of the anatomy of the single vertebra, will give instructions to the students on how to build the epidural region, adding the ligaments and other adjacent tissues until a 3D model is obtained, from the skin to the dural sac. The module is based on the principle of "learning by doing," which is one of the basic principles of adult learning.

## 1.3 Examples of Materials Needed for each Student (Figs. 1 and 2)

A model of three 3B Scientific A76/8 PVC lumbar vertebrae, available online
A closed-cell black neoprene tube for covering and insulating hydraulic pipes
An elastic silicone material, available, for example, among packaging materials
A transparent plastic film for food-type paper
An electrical cable containing some wires inside
A rubber or para tube, such as a surgical drainage tube or similar
A plastic insulating tape
Scissors

After having illustrated in detail the anatomy of the single lumbar vertebra and the anatomical relationships of the lumbar vertebrae with each other and with the entire spine, the construction of the model begins, starting with the ligamentum flavum, represented by a silicone cube that will be adapted by the student and modeled on the interlaminar foramen (Fig. 3). After this, the interspinous ligament will

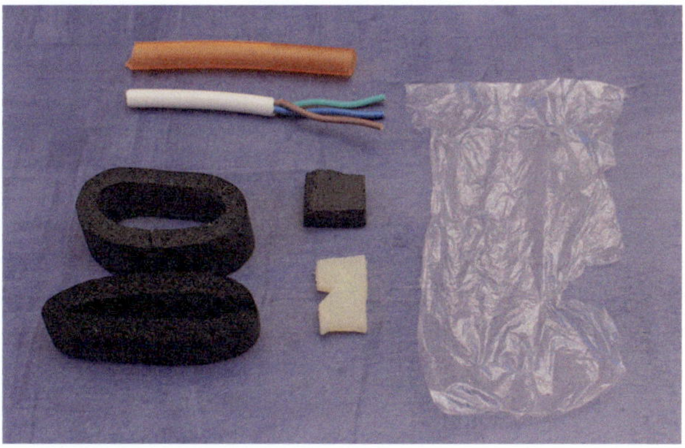

**Fig. 1** Materials needed for the construction of the epidural region model

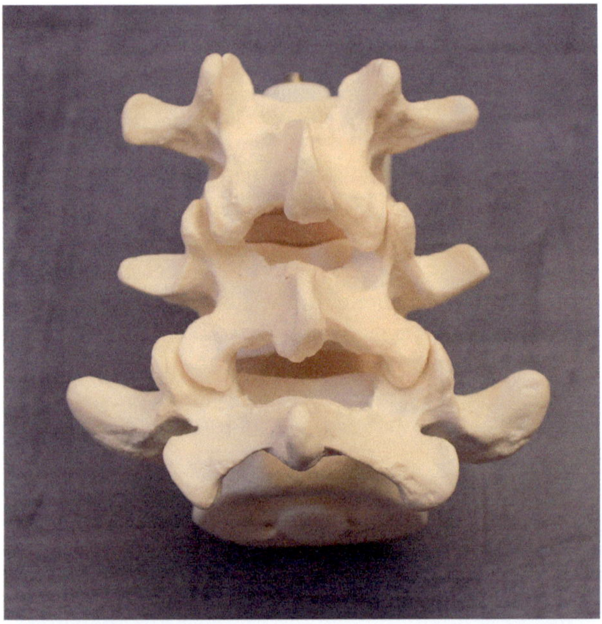

**Fig. 2** The 1:1 scale model of the lumbar vertebrae used for the construction of the epidural region model

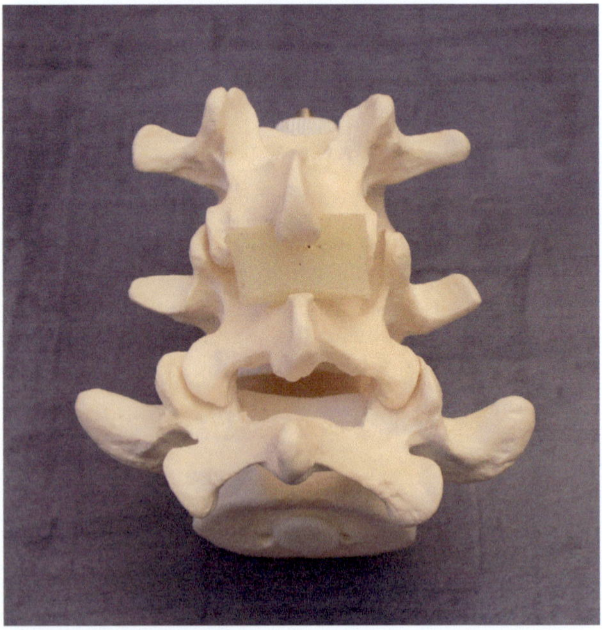

**Fig. 3** The model of the lumbar vertebrae with the inserted silicone cube representing the ligamentum flavum. The student is invited to cut the silicone material to adapt it to the interlaminar foramen

be inserted, represented by a square cut from the neoprene tube, which is low density and represents the interspinous ligament (Fig. 4) and completed with the application of an insulating tape fixed above the spinous processes, to represent the supraspinous ligament, which has a higher density (Fig. 5). Two appropriately sized

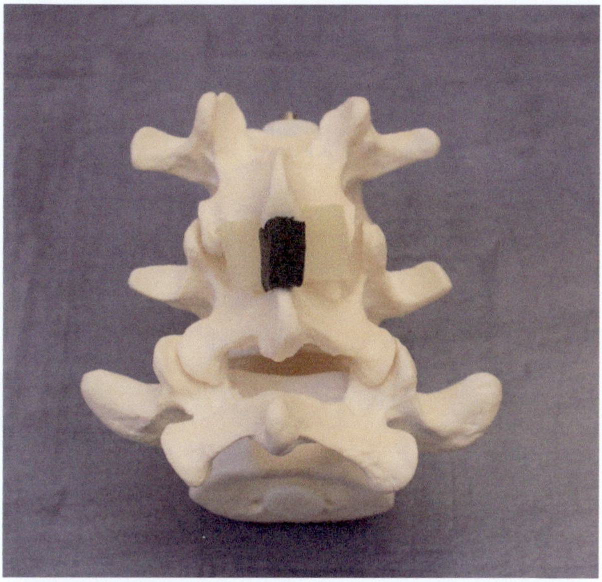

**Fig. 4** The model of the lumbar vertebrae with the inserted neoprene material representing the interspinous ligament

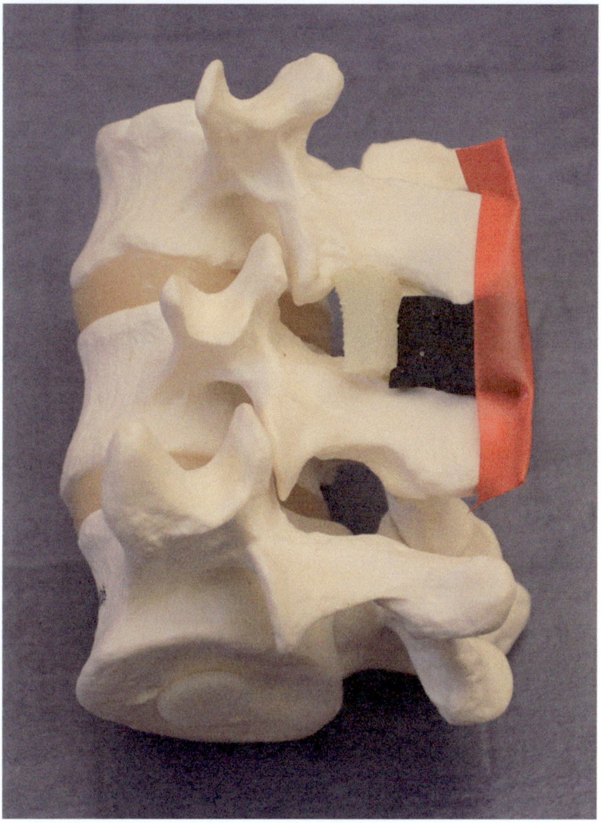

**Fig. 5** A piece of insulating tape (red) is adhered to the spinous processes to represent the supraspinous ligament

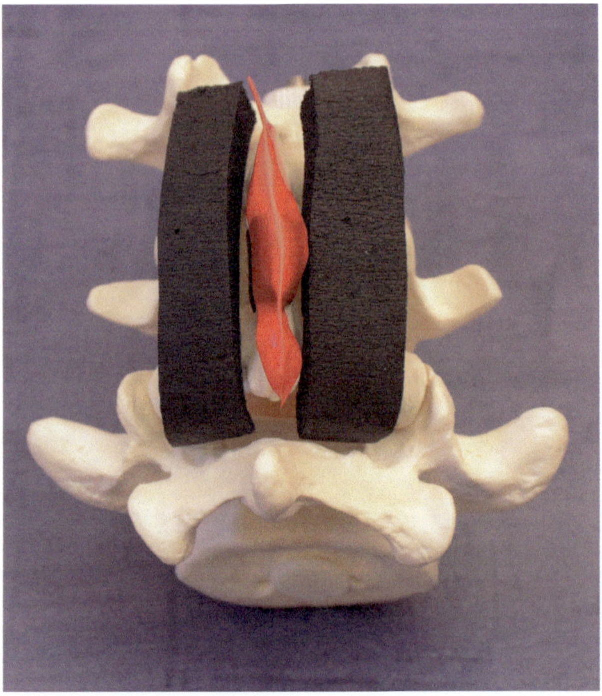

**Fig. 6** Two strips of neoprene are inserted next to the transverse processes to represent the multifidus spinal muscles

cutouts of neoprene will then be inserted on the sides of the model, matching the laminae, to represent the spinal multifidus muscles (Figs. 6 and 7).

Above the model, you can wrap some plastic transparent paper, to represent the skin layer (Fig. 8). The model can be further completed by inserting a rubber tube inside the vertebral canal to simulate the dural sac (Figs. 9 and 10), and once completed, it can be the subject of discussion and observation of the anatomical relationships between the dural sac and the bony canal, as well as easily illustrating to the students the spaces left free by the dural sac inside the bony canal itself, which will be occupied posteriorly and laterally by the epidural fat. Inside the dural sac (the rubber tube), you can insert an electrical cable representing the spinal cord with the spinal roots (Fig. 11), which can in turn be wrapped in a sheet of plastic transparent paper representing the arachnoid membranes. This will allow the tutor to visually explain how the arachnoid membranes surround each individual spinal root inside the dural sac and help the student understand these important anatomical relationships even before having viewed them with slides on a cadaveric model.

After constructing the epidural model, the teacher proceeds with a lesson on anatomy using slides that illustrate the anatomical aspects of the lumbar epidural region with 3D reconstructions and macro- and microphotographs from cadavers or living subjects (MRI images, epiduroscopy, etc.).

At the end of this module, most students begin to discover that anatomy is more complex than they thought and that their knowledge has been enriched by the "integrated anatomical-functional-applicative approach to the block technique."

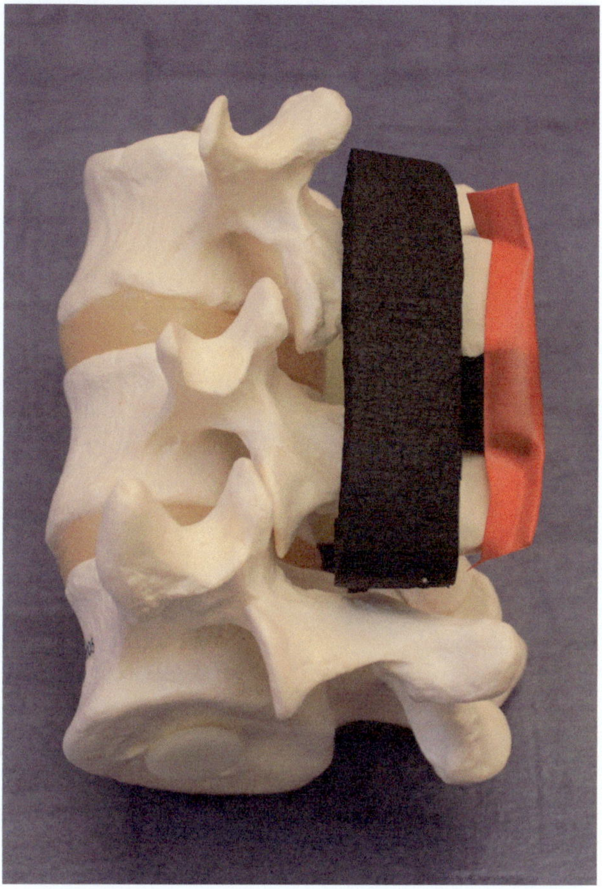

**Fig. 7** The nearly completed model viewed from the side

In particular, the main and most frequent "discoveries" of the students are:

1. The definition of ligaments not as separate and independent entities, but as a supra-interspinous ligament complex, which is an extension of the thoracolumbar fascia.
2. The particular anatomical relationship between the two key elements for the success of the block, the vertebral arch and the ligamentum flavum, and how the latter is distributed on the bony laminae.
3. The fact that there are two ligamenta flava and the occasional presence of a median hiatus.
4. The functions of the epidural fat.
5. The different distribution of epidural fat in various compartments.
6. The anatomy of the dural cuff and the topography of the nerve roots within the lumbar epidural region.
7. The dimensions of the ligaments and the depth of the epidural space, in relation to the distance at which the needle can be pushed inside it.

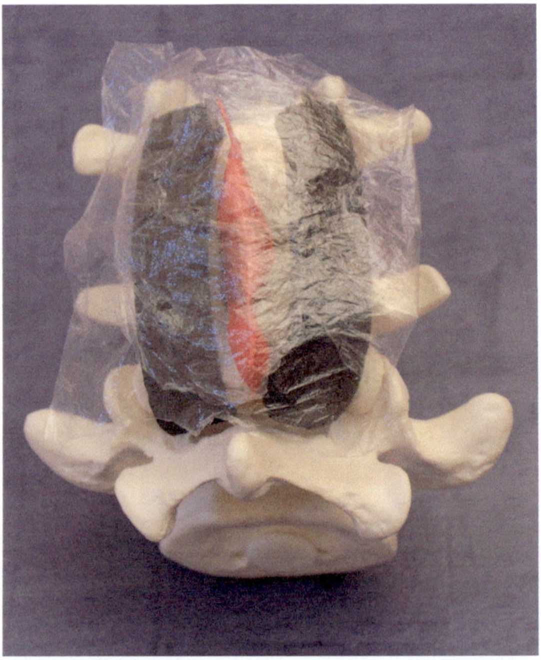

**Fig. 8** The model is completed by wrapping it with transparent plastic paper representing the skin layer

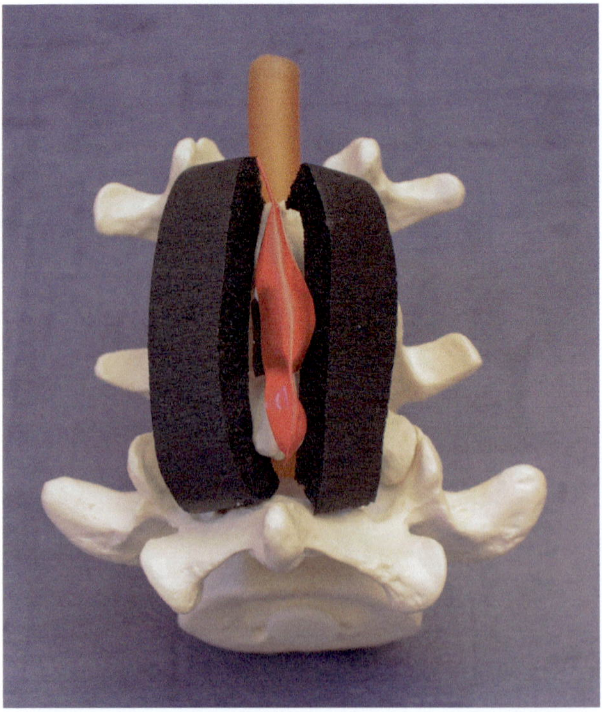

**Fig. 9** A rubber tube is inserted into the vertebral canal to represent the dural sac

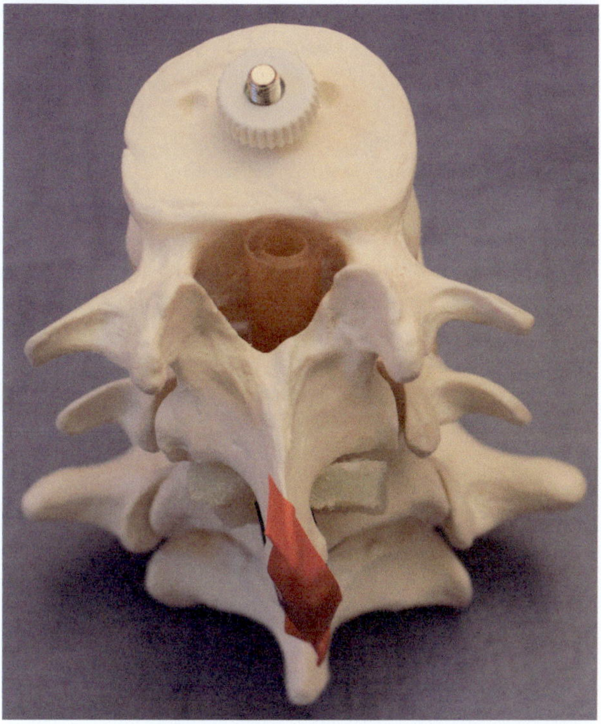

**Fig. 10** A rubber tube is inserted into the vertebral canal to represent the dural sac (view from above)

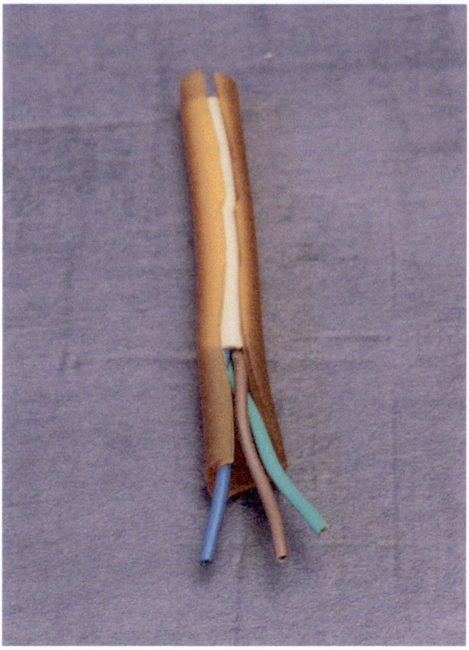

**Fig. 11** An electrical cable is inserted into the rubber tube, which in turn contains electrical wires representing the spinal cord and spinal roots

8. The structure, distribution, and topographic relationships of the meninges (dura and arachnoid).
9. The structure of the arachnoid membranes.
10. The relationship between the arachnoid membranes and the spinal roots, as an explanation for possible failures of spinal anesthesia.
11. The topographic anatomy of the spinal roots in relation to the patient's posture.

This module ends with a summary by the students of what they have learned.

It would also be appropriate for students to write the following questions in their notebooks and try to answer them by listing at least one of the required elements:

What have I consolidated? (List the things I already knew)
What have I learned that is new? (List the things I did not know)
What did I not understand?
What do I want to explore further? (List the things I would like to explore better at home)

After writing the answers, the teacher asks if any of the students want to share their answers with the group.

## 2 Module 2: General Principles

*Everything must be learned not to show off, but to use it. (Lichtenberg)*

### 2.1 Familiarization with the Materials

The teacher introduces the materials for the epidural block.

Each learner has at their disposal a Tuohy needle with introducer, wings, an epidural catheter, an LOR (loss of resistance) syringe, a filter, a connector, a syringe, and a vial of saline solution and is invited to familiarize themselves with the provided materials, observing the details, connections, and measurements (Figs. 12, 13, 14, 15 and 16).

Subsequently, the teacher presents the various models of needles and catheters available on the market, highlighting the common parts, similarities, and differences.

The nomenclature of the individual parts of the materials, their origin, and a brief historical overview can also be clarified.

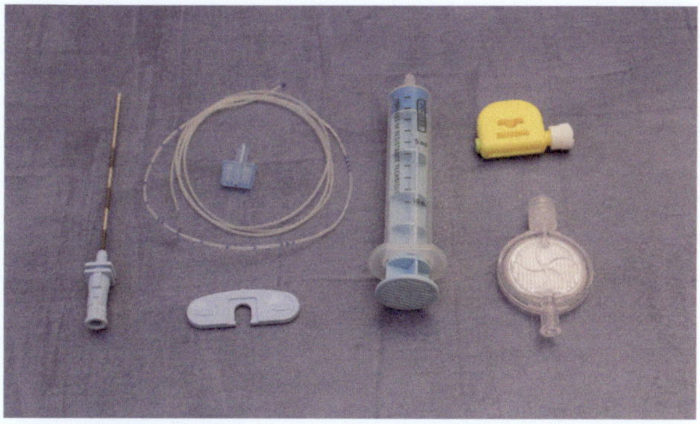

**Fig. 12** Materials used for the epidural block

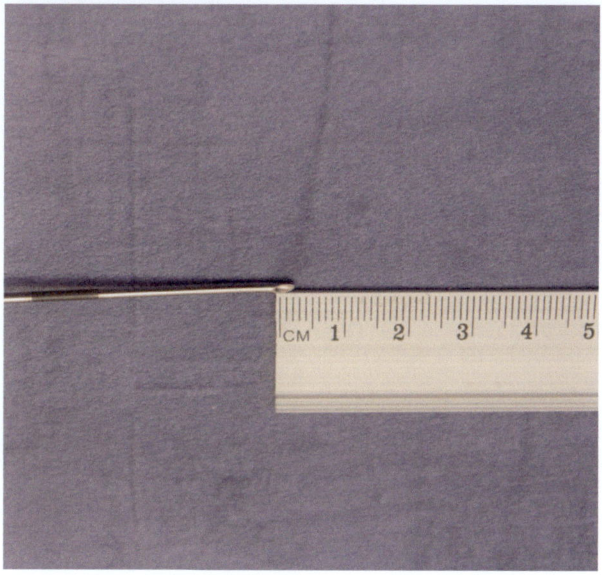


**Fig. 13** Familiarization with the measurements of the bevel of an epidural needle

## 2.2 Familiarization with the General Principles of the Loss of Resistance Technique

*You cannot lose what you have not yet acquired.*

At this stage, the focus is exclusively on recognizing the increase in resistance (ligamentum flavum) and the loss of resistance (epidural space).

Although young trainees are usually eager to try the technique in practice, it is important for the teacher to insist first on the general principles. Usually, most students have already heard about the loss of resistance technique (LORT), but they do not know its principles or origin in detail.

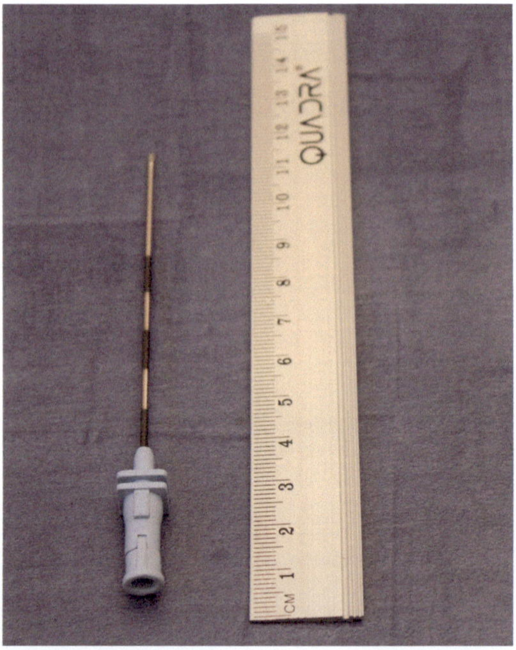


**Fig. 14** Familiarization with the measurements of an epidural needle

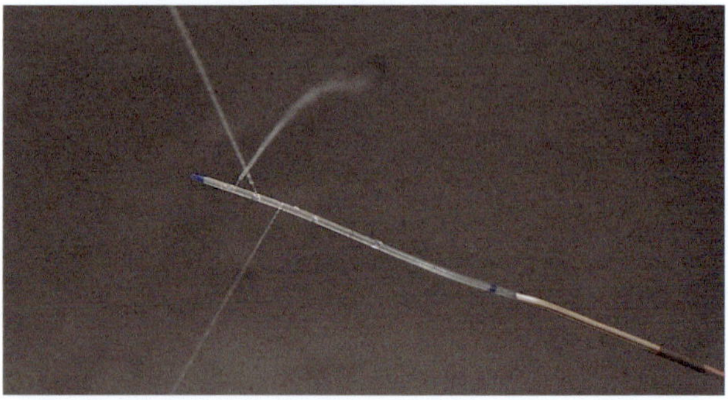

**Fig. 15** Familiarization with the presence of helical holes on the tip of the epidural catheter

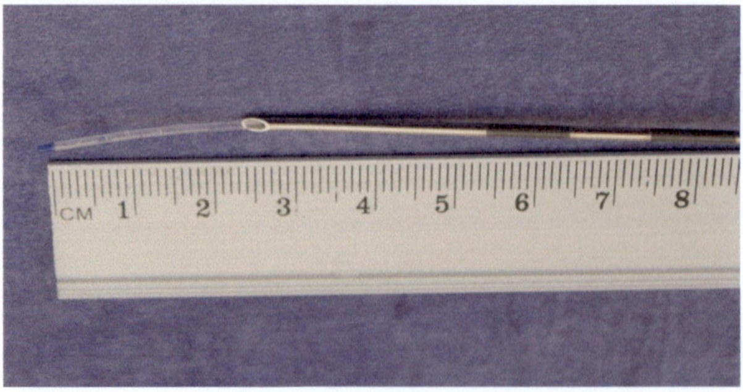


**Fig. 16** Familiarization with the measurements of the epidural catheter

The teacher explains the reasons for using *LORT* in lumbar epidural, mentioning the existence of other techniques for thoracic and cervical epidural (not covered in this course).

The fundamental concepts to be acquired at this stage of learning are as follows:

1. "You cannot lose what you have not yet acquired," so before looking for a loss of resistance, you must focus on finding the increase in resistance, offered by the ligamentum flavum when it encounters the needle.
2. The differences in density of the various tissues crossed by the needle cannot be perceived if the needle is introduced too quickly or intermittently, so the needle must be inserted continuously, constantly, and slowly.
3. The needle-syringe-filled-with-liquid system is incompressible if the needle's bevel is closed (by the ligamentum flavum), so the pressure on the piston will advance the system, which in turn will automatically stop as soon as the needle's bevel is open again (in the epidural space).

This module is also based on the principle of "learning by doing," so using a Tuohy needle, an *LOR* syringe filled with saline, and a silicone cube, the teacher explains the general principles of increasing and losing resistance (Fig. 17). This explanation is followed by practical exercises by the students.

During this exercise, the teacher can have the students experience the advantages of a slow, constant, and continuous technique vs intermittent techniques by practicing the "overshooting" phenomenon (protrusion from the silicone cube).

Like the previous module, this module also ends with a summary by the students of what they have learned and the written answers to the three end-of-session questions (What have I consolidated? What have I learned that is new? What do I want to explore further?) followed by sharing the answers.

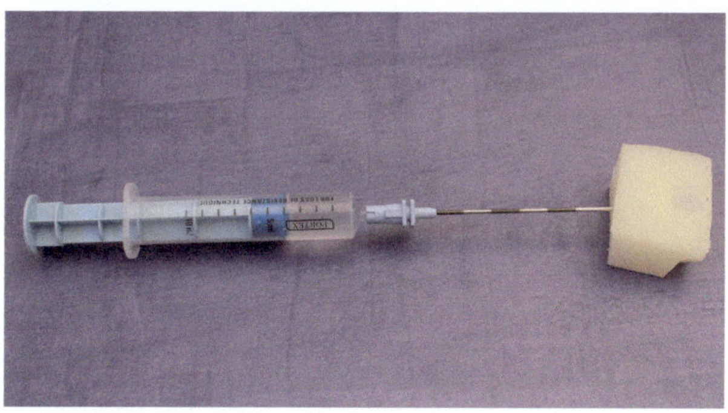

**Fig. 17** Material used for explaining the general principles of loss of resistance

## 3 Module 3: Fundamentals with the Simulator

*Epidural in Four Moves* (Fig. 18)

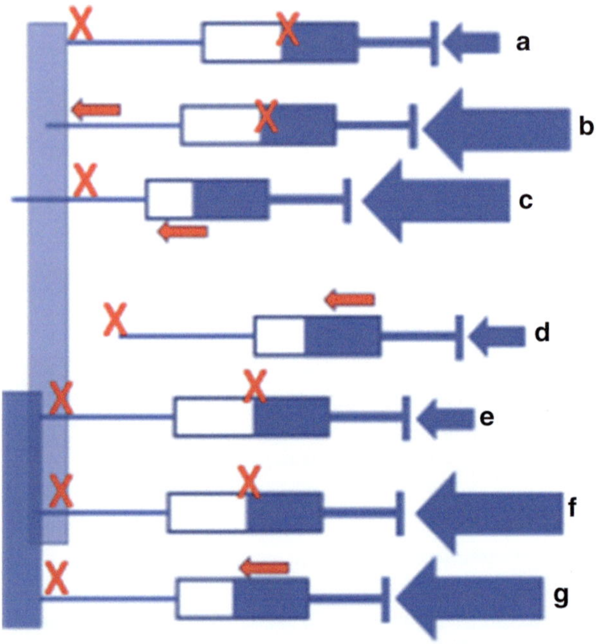


**Fig. 18** (a) If the needle is inserted into the ligamentum flavum and slight pressure is applied to the plunger, the piston does not move because the needle tip is closed by the ligament. (b) By increasing the pressure on the plunger in a continuous, constant, but decisive manner, the needle progresses through the tissues against resistance. Observe that the needle slowly penetrates the tissues while the piston remains stationary. (c) By pushing progressively and constantly on the piston when the needle is in the ligamentum flavum, as soon as the needle tip reaches the epidural space, the piston is suddenly and unequivocally pushed forward, releasing the saline solution into the epidural space. At the same time, the needle's progression automatically stops. (d) If the needle is *not* inserted into the ligamentum flavum and slight pressure is applied to the plunger, the piston moves forward because the needle tip is not closed by the inextensible yellow ligament, but by the soft tissues that are easily infiltrated by water. (e) By applying slight pressure to the plunger, the piston does not move because the needle tip is inserted into the ligamentum flavum in the portion where it attaches to the bone (vertebral arch). (f) By increasing the pressure on the plunger in a continuous, constant, but decisive manner, the needle does *not* progress through the tissues against resistance. Please observe that the needle does *not* slowly penetrate the tissues while the piston remains stationary. Feel the sensation of invincible resistance. The needle tip is on the vertebral arch. (g) By applying slight pressure on the plunger, the piston moves because the needle tip is against the bone, so resistance may be lost. However, by increasing the pressure on the plunger in a continuous, constant, but firm manner, the needle does *not* progress through the tissues against resistance. Observe that the needle does *not* slowly penetrate the tissues while the piston remains stationary. Feel the sensation of invincible resistance. The needle tip is on the vertebral arch

In this module, students are divided into small groups, to give everyone the opportunity to practice multiple times. The P61 epidural simulator from 3B Scientific containing the Epidural Module$^{EESOA}$ (see Chap. "Epidural Simulators") is used for the exercise.

In this phase, the simulator is used exclusively as an object through which the Tuohy needle is passed to appreciate and recognize the differences in resistance offered by the encountered tissues. It should be clarified to the students that the purpose of this module is to acquire the tactile sensitivity necessary to recognize the different densities of the tissues that the epidural needle may encounter during its path to reach the epidural space.

Each student is then invited to sit in front of the simulator, choose an interspinous space, and insert the Tuohy needle with a slow and constant movement, stopping only when they believe they have perceived an increase in resistance to the needle's advancement and connecting the syringe (filled with liquid) to the needle.

**Move 1: Recognize the Increase in Resistance (Ligamentum Flavum)**
If the needle is inserted into the ligamentum flavum, applying slight pressure on the plunger, the piston does not move because the needle tip is closed by the ligament. By increasing the pressure on the plunger in a continuous, constant, but decisive manner, the needle progresses through the tissues against resistance. Observe that the needle slowly penetrates the tissues while the piston remains stationary.

**Move 2: Recognize the Loss of Resistance (Epidural Space)**
By pushing progressively and constantly on the piston when the needle is in the ligamentum flavum, as soon as the needle tip reaches the epidural space, the piston is suddenly and unequivocally pushed forward, suddenly discharging the saline solution into the epidural space. Simultaneously, the needle's progression automatically stops.

**Move 3: Recognize the False Loss of Resistance**
If the needle is *not* inserted into the ligamentum flavum, applying slight pressure on the plunger, the piston moves forward because the needle tip is not closed by the inextensible ligamentum flavum, but by the soft tissues that are easily infiltrated by water.

**Move 4: Recognize the False Increase in Resistance or False Loss of Resistance Due to Bone Contact**

(a) Applying slight pressure on the plunger, the piston does not move because the needle tip is inserted into the ligamentum flavum in its portion where it attaches to the bone (vertebral arch). By increasing the pressure on the plunger in a continuous, constant, but decisive manner, the needle does *not* progress through the tissues against resistance. Observe that the needle does *not* slowly penetrate the tissues while the piston remains stationary. Feel the sensation of invincible resistance.

(b) Applying slight pressure on the plunger, the piston moves because the needle tip is against the bone, so resistance can be lost. However, by increasing the pressure on the plunger in a continuous, constant, but decisive manner, the needle does *not* progress through the tissues against resistance. Observe that the needle does *not* slowly penetrate the tissues while the piston remains stationary. Feel the sensation of invincible resistance.

**Problem-Solving**

**Move 3**. In the case of identification of a false loss of resistance, the student is invited to advance the needle slowly by a few millimeters without applying pressure on the piston, stop the needle, and retry until the perceived resistance has the characteristics described in moves 1 and 2.

In this way, the students get used to working in successive logical steps, with an algorithmic procedure that accustoms them to reflect on the diagnosis (where the needle might be) rather than injecting large amounts of fluid without first having an idea of the topographical relationships of the needle tip with the tissues crossed.

**Bone Contact: Differential Diagnosis and Door Jamb Principle**

In the case of bone contact (move 4), the fundamental steps that the student must learn are the following:

**Problem-Solving for Move 4a:**

1. Resistance can also be lost against the bone: if the needle bevel is directly in contact with the bone, the needle tip is open and it is therefore possible, by pressing on the plunger, to inject the fluid. Obviously, in this case, there is no simultaneous advancement of the needle. This can be easily demonstrated to students using the vertebral model, placing the needle against any bone surface (preferably the vertebral arch) and showing how the fluid can be easily injected onto the bone, thanks to the curved nature of the needle bevel.
2. The loss of resistance on the bone can occur both deeply and superficially. In the case of inserting the needle a few centimeters from the skin (Fig. 19), it can be

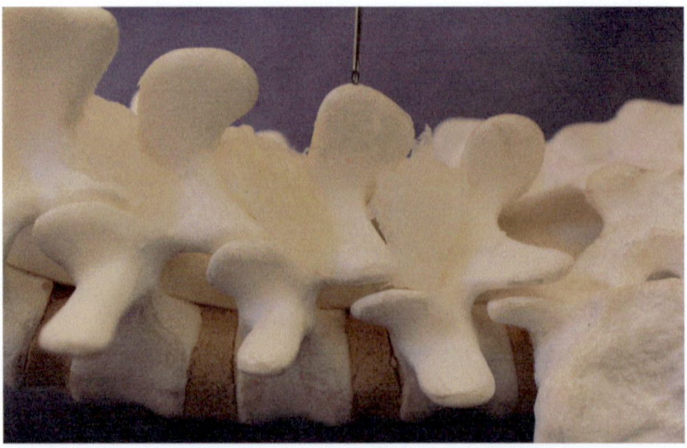

**Fig. 19** Demonstration with the model of a superficial bone contact (apophysis)

suspected that the needle has met a spinous process or a superficial portion of the vertebra, and therefore, the needle will need to be reinserted and the chosen space for its insertion reevaluated.

If, on the other hand, the needle has been inserted more deeply, it can be reasonably assumed that the bone resistance we have perceived is due to the contact between the needle and the lamina of the vertebral arch (Fig. 20). In this case, the maneuver to be performed will be to check the patient's position. Probably, the spine has accidentally rotated, exposing the bone lamina to the operator. The student thus learns that for each "diagnosis," there is a "therapy" and that not all bone contacts have the same origin and therefore are not resolved in the same way.

**Problem-Solving for Move 4b:**

Using the vertebral model (prepared with a layer of silicone to simulate the ligamentum flavum), the teacher invites the student to observe that the needle can be correctly inserted into the ligamentum flavum, but in its portion where it adheres to the bone lamina (Fig. 21). This is why the subsequent pressure of the operator on the syringe plunger does not achieve the loss of resistance, despite having correctly

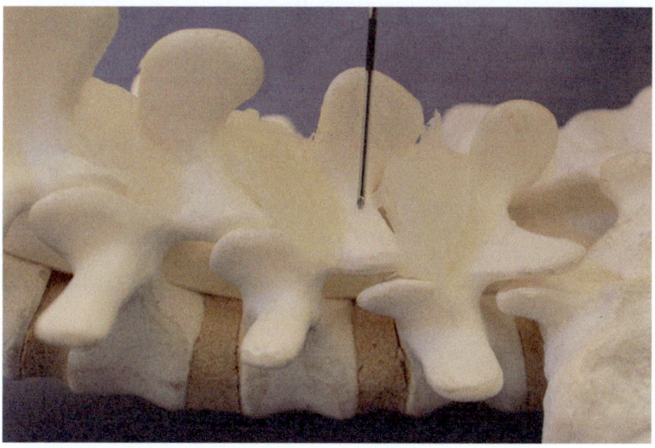

**Fig. 20** Demonstration with the model of a deep bone contact directly on the vertebral arch

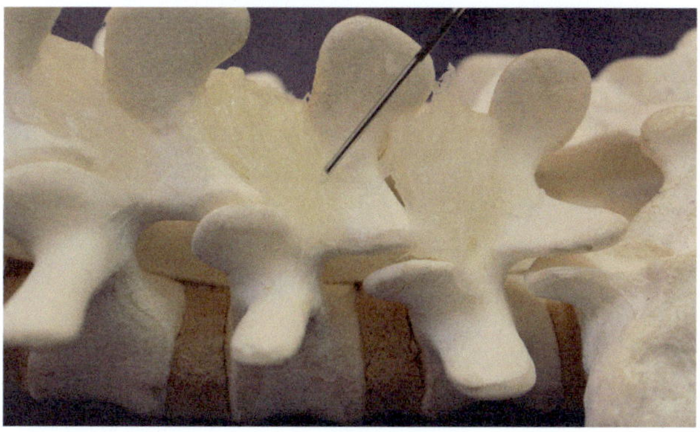

**Fig. 21** Demonstration with the model of a deep bone contact on the vertebral arch mediated by the ligamentum flavum

perceived, just before, the sensation of increased resistance typical of the ligamentum flavum. In this case, the solution to this technical problem is completely different from the previous cases and is based on the technique we have called the "door jamb and four quadrants maneuver." We have indeed compared the needle placed in the portion of the ligamentum flavum that inserts onto the bone lamina to the hand of a subject who, in the dark, must explore an unknown room in order to exit. The subject will cautiously "grope" by touching the wall until he identifies the door jamb with his touch: at this point, he stops because he knows that in two moves, he will find the door (either to his right or to his left). Similarly, the anesthetist, having inserted the needle into the portion of the ligamentum flavum inserted on the vertebral arch (after perceiving an invincible resistance and noting the depth of the needle), will have four moves available to reach the epidural space, directing the needle in the medial, lateral, cranial, and caudal directions. The four-quadrant maneuver must be performed slowly, advancing the needle millimetrically and always checking its position at each small advancement in one of the four directions, using pressure on the plunger, observing if the needle begins to progress and subsequently entering the epidural space. The maneuver should be taught using the "four hands" technique (Sect. 3.1) in which both the teacher and the student perform the technique together on the simulator. The same technique will be used later on the real patient. The advantage of using it first on the simulator makes the student more familiar and confident with this technique before it is put into practice on the real patient in environmental conditions that are certainly very different and often more stressful.

## 3.1 Four Hands Technique on the Simulator

The "four hands" technique involves two phases. In the first phase, the tutor performs the technique with the student's hands on his; in the second phase, the student performs the technique with the tutor placing his hands on the student's hands. In this way, the tutor can not only perceive what the student is perceiving during the execution of the technique but also has the possibility to control and direct the "needle-syringe-student's hands system," guiding it passively or actively when necessary. The technique can be performed with the simulator, but also, subsequently, on the patient.

**Phase 1** The student's hands (wearing blue gloves in the figures) are on the tutor's hands (wearing white gloves in the figures). The tutor performs the technique, explaining step by step the movements they are making and reporting to the student the sensations that the needle passing through the tissues transmits to their fingers.

The student places their thumb on the tutor's thumb as the needle is inserted (Fig. 22). During the loss of resistance maneuver, the student can place his fingers only on the plunger to appreciate the sensation of loss of resistance (Fig. 23) or simultaneously on the plunger and the needle to appreciate the advancement of the needle and the loss of resistance (Fig. 24).

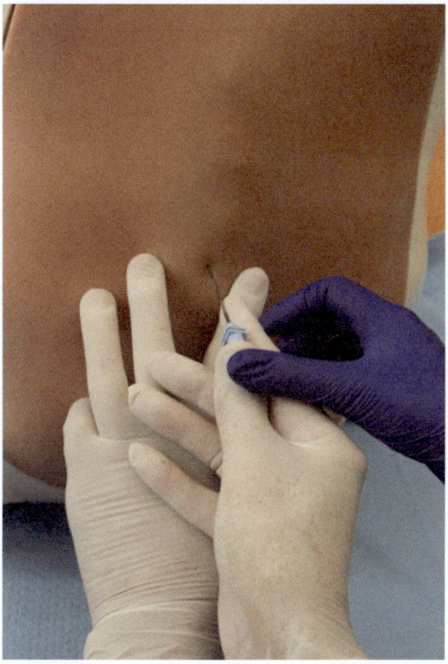

**Fig. 22** Four-handed technique. Phase 1: the student's hands (blue gloves) are on the tutor's hands (white gloves) who performs the technique, explaining step by step the movements being executed and reporting to the student the sensations that the needle passing through the tissues transmits to their fingers

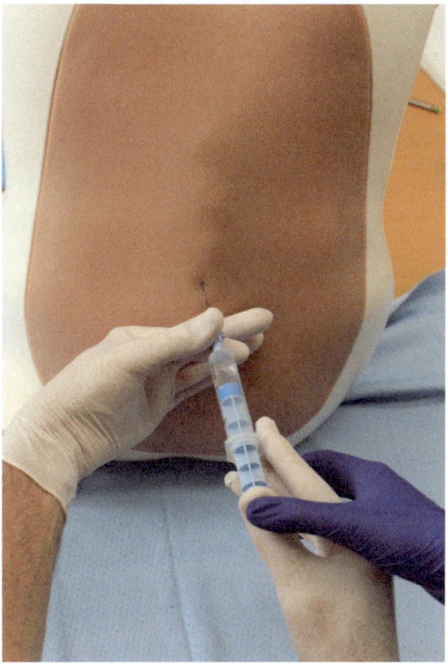

**Fig. 23** Four-handed technique. Phase 1: the student's hands (blue gloves) are on the tutor's hands (white gloves). The student places their thumb on the tutor's thumb while the needle is inserted. During the loss of resistance maneuver, the student can place their fingers on the piston to appreciate the sensation of loss of resistance

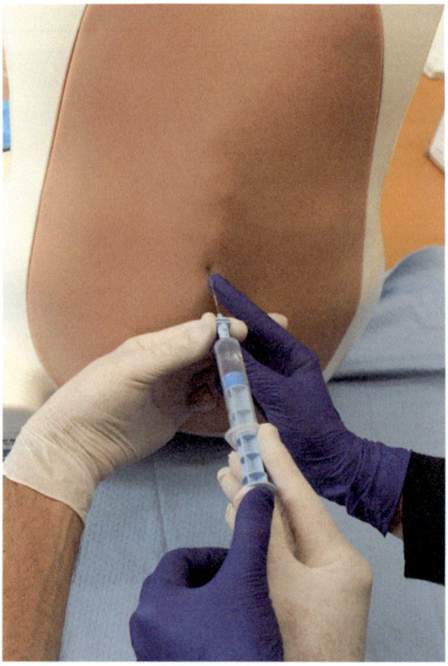

**Fig. 24** Four-handed technique. Phase 1: the student's hands (blue gloves) are on the tutor's hands (white gloves). During the loss of resistance maneuver, the student can place their fingers simultaneously on the piston and the needle to appreciate the needle's advancement and the loss of resistance

**Phase 2** The tutor's hands (wearing white gloves in the figures) are on the student's hands (wearing blue gloves in the figures) who performs the technique.

During the needle insertion maneuver, the tutor places his finger on the needle hub to perceive the same sensations that the needle transmits to the student's fingers during its progression through the underlying tissues (Fig. 25).

During the loss of resistance maneuver, the tutor's dominant hand controls the advancement of the plunger while a finger of the other hand placed on the needle appreciates its progression without obstructing the student's view (Fig. 26). Note the position of the tutor's thumb, which is gently placed on the student's thumb, and the position of the index and middle fingers, which are ready to block the student's attempts to advance the plunger, if and when necessary.

Alternatively, and when the student is a little more experienced, the tutor may decide to place only his thumb on the plunger during the student's advancement of the needle-syringe system (Fig. 27). The detail of the tutor's finger position is indicated in Fig. 28.

In the event that the needle is inserted into the ligamentum flavum, but in its portion where it adheres to the bone plate, the technique we have called the "four quadrants maneuver" can be performed together. The tutor grasps the needle cone with the fingers of his nondominant hand, firmly overlapping those of the student, and simultaneously grips the syringe plunger as in the previous maneuvers (Fig. 29). In this way, he can actively direct the needle tip, leaving the student the role of passively following the movement (Fig. 30).

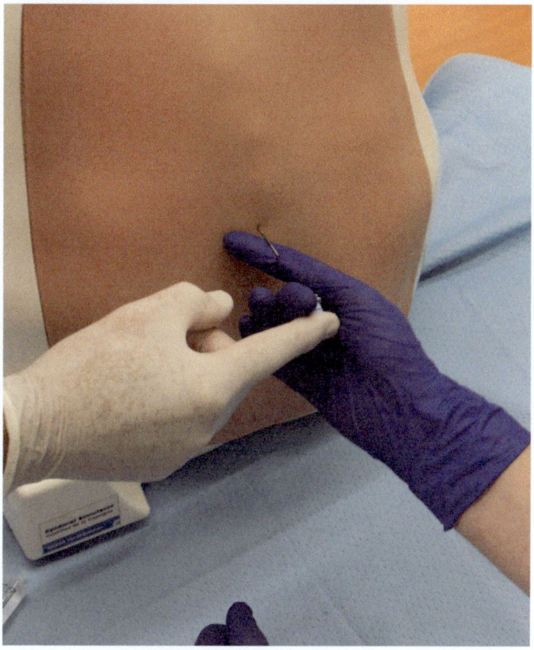

**Fig. 25** Four-handed technique. Phase 2: the tutor's hands (white gloves) are on the student's hands (blue gloves) who performs the technique. During the needle insertion maneuver, the tutor places their finger on the needle hub to perceive the same sensations that the needle transmits to the student's fingers during its progression through the underlying tissues

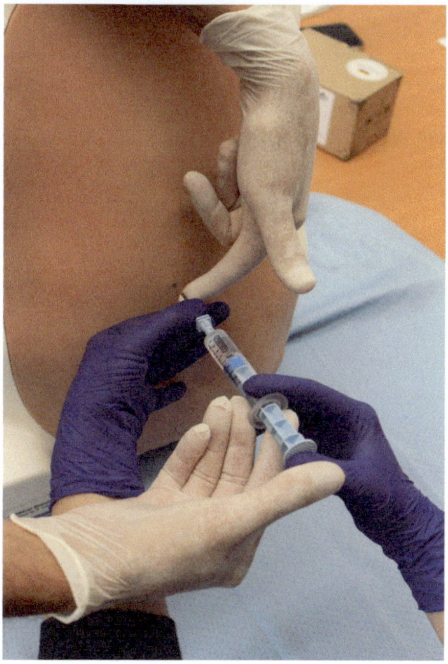

**Fig. 26** Four-handed technique. Phase 2: the tutor's hands (white gloves) are on the student's hands (blue gloves) who performs the technique. During the loss of resistance maneuver, the tutor's dominant hand controls the piston's advancement while a finger from the other hand placed on the needle appreciates its progression without obstructing the student's view

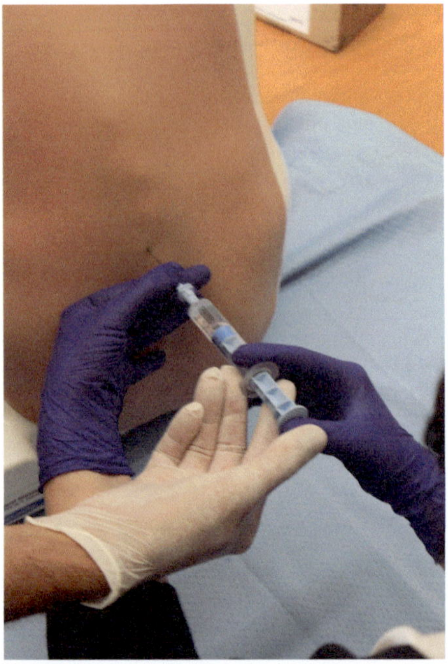

**Fig. 27** Four-handed technique. Phase 2: the tutor's hands (white gloves) are on the student's hands (blue gloves) who performs the technique. Notice the position of the tutor's thumb, which is gently placed on the student's thumb, and the position of the index and middle fingers, which are ready to block the student's attempts to advance the piston, if and when necessary

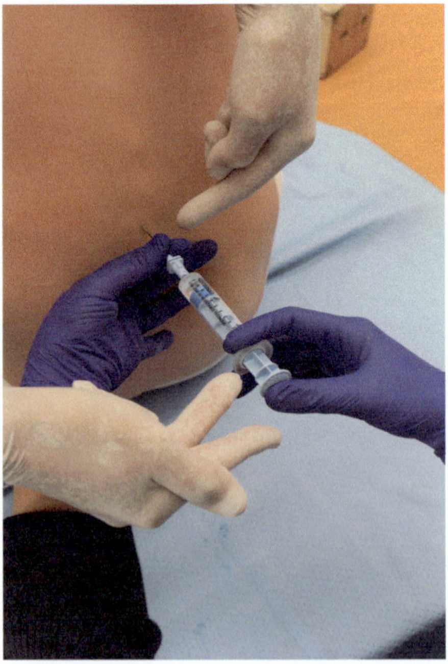

**Fig. 28** Four-handed technique. Phase 2: the tutor's hands (white gloves) are on the student's hands (blue gloves) who performs the technique. Detail of the tutor's fingers' position

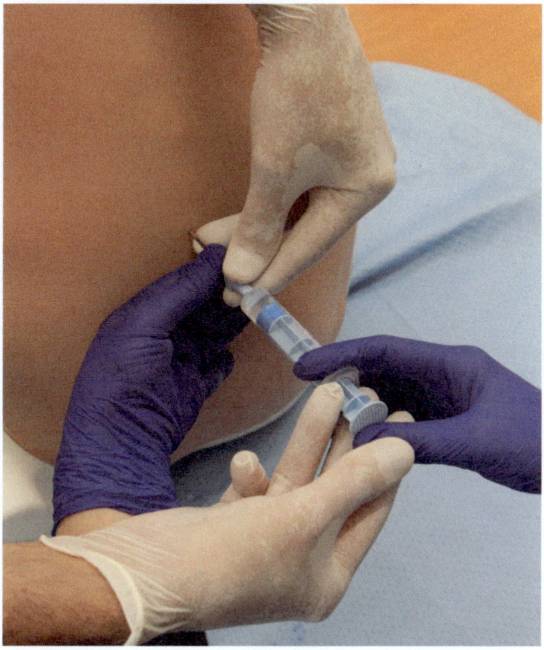

**Fig. 29** Four-handed technique. Phase 2: the tutor's hands (white gloves) are on the student's hands (blue gloves) who is performing the technique. "Four quadrants" maneuver: the tutor grasps the needle cone with the fingers of their nondominant hand, firmly overlapping the student's fingers, and simultaneously grips the syringe plunger as in the previous maneuvers

When the student has reached sufficient competence, it will be enough for the tutor to gently rest his finger on the needle shaft, to perceive the sensations elicited by the passage of the needle through the tissues and transmitted to the needle itself, which will thus be perceived simultaneously by the student and tutor (Fig. 31).

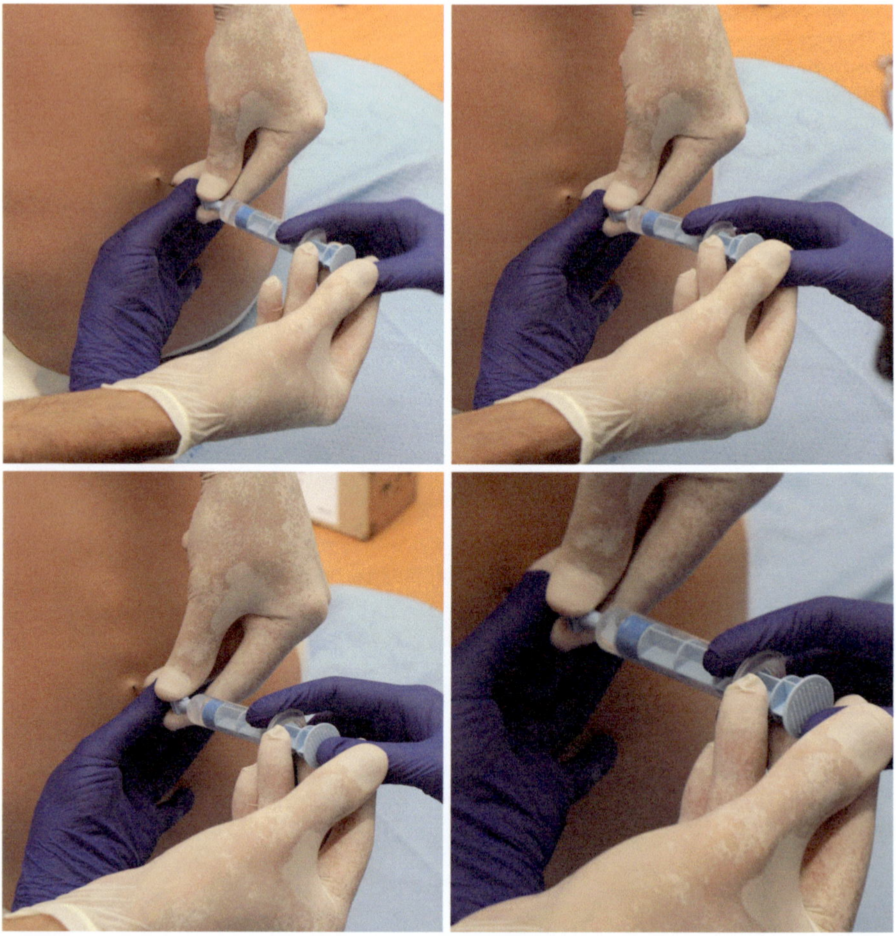

**Fig. 30** Four-handed technique. Phase 2: the tutor's hands (white gloves) are on the student's hands (blue gloves) who is performing the technique. "Four quadrants" maneuver: the tutor actively directs the needle tip, leaving the student with the role of passively following the movement

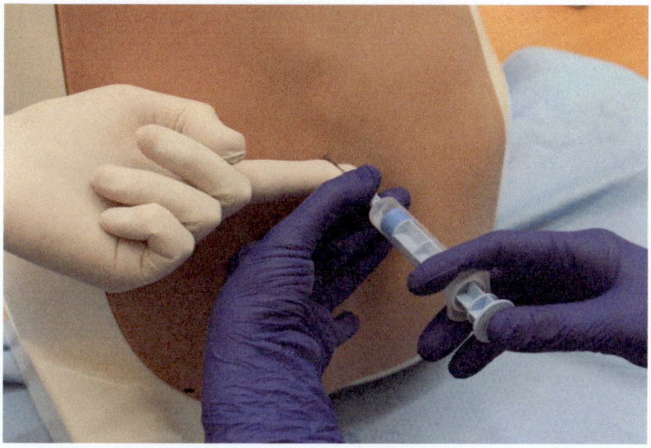

**Fig. 31** When the student has reached sufficient competence, the tutor gently rests their finger on the needle shaft to perceive the sensations elicited by the passage of the needle through the tissues and transmitted to the needle itself, which will thus be perceived simultaneously by the student and tutor

## 4 Module 4: See and Hear What Is Perceived with the CompuFlo-Trainer

*Four moves seen and heard*

This module is optional as it requires the CompuFlo instrument, so if you do not have the instrument, you can proceed directly to the execution of module 5.

The CompuFlo instrument (Milestone Scientific Inc., Livingston, NJ, USA) is able to measure in real time the pressure of human tissues at the tip of a needle [1] (Fig. 32).

This system is unique as the pressure constitutes a feedback circuit and a system controller, thus regulating the electromechanical motor that controls the flow and fluid dispensed by the system. This instrument has been studied and validated for epidural use both for its routine use and in difficult cases [2–4] and can distinguish the false loss of resistance due to the position of the epidural needle within the tissues of the epidural region and the true loss of resistance due to the penetration of the needle into the epidural space [5].

Furthermore, the CompuFlo instrument has proven to be an objective tool for teaching epidural block to trainees using an epidural simulator [6, 7].

This exercise can be used at any time during training, both in the initial phase and later, after the student has performed a certain number of blocks on the real patient, to consolidate (acoustically and visually) the steps and understanding of the technique.

In this module, the simulator is still used exclusively as an object through which the Tuohy needle is passed. The purpose is to appreciate and recognize the differences in resistance offered by the encountered tissues, having the objective feedback of the CompuFlo and comparing the objectivity of the instrument with the quality of one's tactile perception.

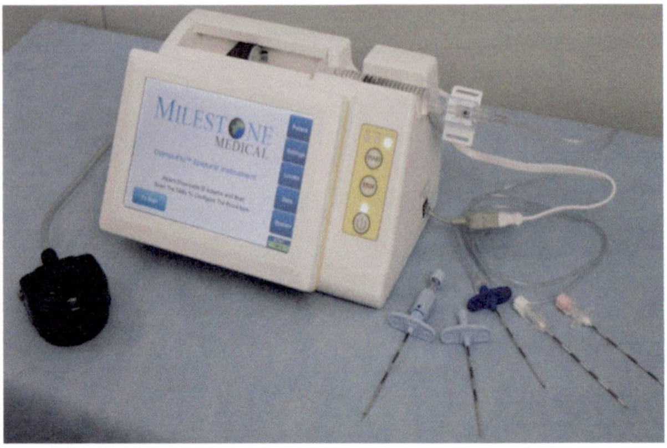


**Fig. 32** The CompuFlo device for identifying the epidural space

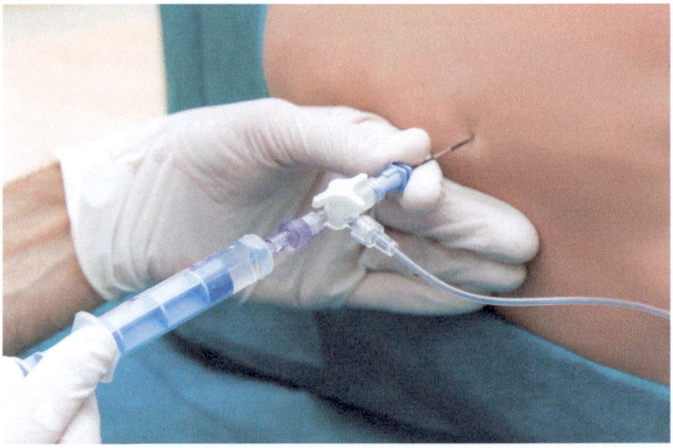

**Fig. 33** Detail of the connection of the CompuFlo with a three-way tap, an anti-reflux valve, and a loss of resistance syringe filled with saline solution

After explaining the general principles of operation and analysis of the instrument's graph and acoustics, the exercises of the previous module are repeated with the aid of the CompuFlo.

The device is connected as usual, with the exception that between the Tuohy needle and the connection tube with the device, a three-way stopcock, an anti-reflux valve, and a loss of resistance syringe (LOR syringe) filled with saline solution are inserted (Fig. 33).

The exercise proceeds as follows.

After inserting the needle a few centimeters inside the simulator, connect the needle to the three-way stopcock (leaving the communication needle-syringe-instrument open) connected to the tubing set, which in turn is connected to the device, and invite the student to advance the needle-syringe system very slowly and without interruptions. If the three-way stopcock is kept open while the needle advances, the student can observe on the screen some small increases and decreases in pressure (blue column) accompanied by changes in the sound of the acoustic tone due to the different densities of the tissues crossed by the needle and also the intensity of the pressure applied with the thumb on the syringe plunger.

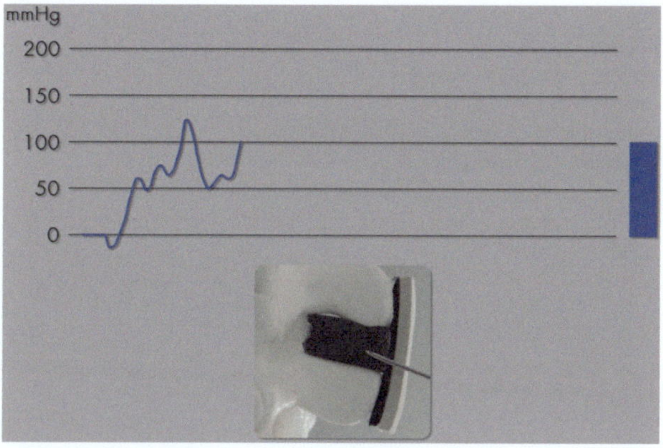


**Fig. 34** When the needle is located somewhere in the soft tissues or the interspinous ligament (false increase/decrease in resistance), the pressure gradually increases but is not be followed by a plateau for more than 5 s (the pressure bar remains blue). Bottom, below the graph: the epidural needle position

After becoming familiar with the system, the student manipulates the three-way stopcock to close communication with the CompuFlo and proceeds with the technique of locating the epidural space using the *LOR* syringe. If at any point in the process there is uncertainty, confusion, or an inconclusive interpretation, the student must stop the needle's advancement and use the CompuFlo tool (connecting the three-way stopcock to the needle and excluding the syringe) to verify the needle's position. This maneuver provides the learner with objective information to distinguish between a true and a false loss of resistance, a bone contact, or to confirm the correct positioning of the needle in the ligamentum flavum or the epidural space.

In fact, once the operator has stopped the needle, there are four possible outcomes corresponding to as many CompuFlo-Trainer patterns:

1. The needle is located somewhere in the soft tissues or the interspinous ligament (false increase/decrease in resistance): in this case, the pressure will gradually increase but will not be followed by a plateau for more than 5 seconds (the pressure bar remains blue) (Fig. 34).

2a. The needle encounters a bone (bone contact): in this case, the pressure and the height of the audible tone increase dramatically and stably (the pressure bar turns red), but the needle cannot advance.

2b. The needle partially encounters the bone (for example, the needle has encountered the vertebral lamina somewhere in the area where the ligamenta flava are inserted on the lamina): in this case, the pressure and the acoustic tone increase dramatically and inconsistently (the pressure bar may turn red), but the needle cannot advance.

3. The needle is located in the ligamentum flavum: in this case, the pressure and the acoustic tone increase dramatically and stably (the pressure bar turns red) and the needle can slowly proceed through the ligament (Fig. 35).

4. The needle is located in the epidural space: in this case, the pressure suddenly and greatly reduces and will be very low, and a stable plateau will be noticed for more than 5 s. The acoustic tone will be low (Fig. 36).

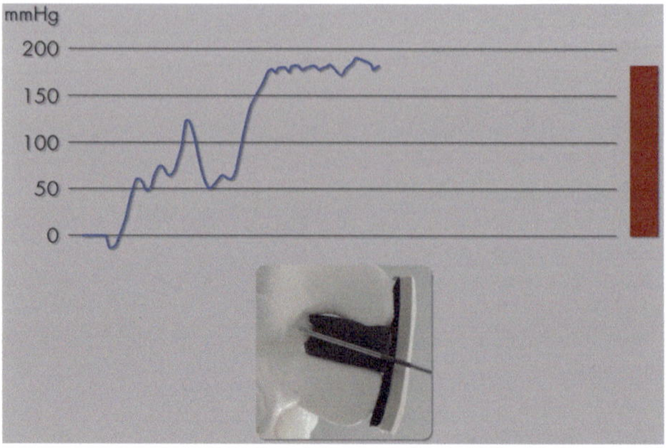


**Fig. 35** When the needle is located in the ligamentum flavum, the pressure and the acoustic tone increase dramatically and stably (the pressure bar turns red). Bottom, below the graph: the epidural needle position

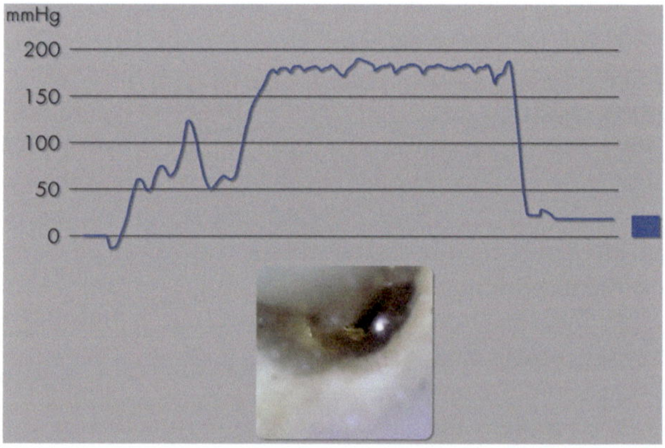


**Fig. 36** When the needle is in the epidural space, the pressure suddenly and greatly reduces, and a stable plateau is noticed for more than 5 s. The acoustic tone is low. Bottom, below the graph: the epidural needle position inside the epidural space (simulator epiduroscopic vision)

A variant provides that the instrument is used as it should be used on the patient, that is, connecting the device directly to the needle and using the CompuFlo to locate the epidural space. In this case, the criteria used to differentiate a true loss of resistance (True-LOR) from the identification of a false loss of resistance (False-LOR) are as follows:

1. A correct loss of resistance, indicating the achievement of the epidural space, is defined as an increase in pressure followed by a sudden and prolonged drop (>5 s) in pressure (usually greater than 50% of the maximum pressure), resulting in the formation of a "low and stable pressure plateau for at least 5 seconds."
2. A false loss of resistance is defined as an increase in pressure followed by a drop in pressure (usually less than 50% of the maximum pressure) that is transient and brief, which is not sustained or not sufficient to represent a "low and stable pressure plateau." If the pressure increases again and quickly after a drop in pressure, this is identified as a false loss of resistance, and the student can decide to continue advancing the needle.

The use of CompuFlo allows the student to compare his tactile sensations with the pressure differences detected by the instrument both fluidly and continuously and intermittently, using the three-way tap.

At the end of the procedure, "the history of the needle's path to the epidural space" can be displayed on the screen or printed and discussed with the instructor.

The added value of using this tool is that it forces (and therefore accustoms) the student to advance the needle very slowly and to appreciate the tactile sensations that change as the needle progresses through the tissues, whether it is the simulated tissue of the simulator or the real patient. For each change in pressure wave and each change in tone of the acoustic signal, there is a modification of the tissue density encountered, and by associating these objective elements with their own tactile sensations, the student experiences and learns to pay attention to even the subtlest differences in tissue density, greatly acquiring or consolidating mastery of the technique.

## 5 Module 5: Problem Setting, or how to Reduce the Complexity of the Technique—Creation of a Checklist and Use of the EMME Video Method

*Using mirror neurons*

This module is carried out on the epidural simulator. The instructor performs the technique proficiently in front of the students, from the introduction of the needle to the insertion of the catheter into the epidural space and the removal of the needle from the skin, preferably in accordance with the checklist used by the school or with the department curriculum.

In this phase, the instructor explains in detail all the steps of the technique, dividing them into various blocks in accordance with the checklist.

To reinforce the learning of this module, we use the projection of the EMME video, which consists of projecting a video that illustrates where to direct the gaze and focus attention while practicing the epidural block (for details see Appendix 1).

In this module, a guided organization of an epidural checklist built by the students is included, which can be based on what they have learned and seen so far. Each student can write down all the steps of the epidural technique, starting from the positioning of the patient to the fixation of the catheter, and share them with the group and the tutor who will complete the missing steps.

Depending on the time available, it may be useful at the end of this module to use complementary techniques such as mentalization (imagining the necessary steps to reach the epidural space), constructing a written sequence, or composing a puzzle (in this case, the various steps of the technique are illustrated/described on pieces of a puzzle [paper or even computerized] that must be reassembled sequentially and chronologically). This work can be done individually or in a group. The session ends with the learning of the epidural checklist that will be used from now on. In the absence of a departmental epidural checklist, validated checklists derived from the literature [8] (Chap. "Assessing Learning", Fig. 5) can be used.

# 6 Module 6: The "Hands-on" Technique: The Proficient Epidural

*No one can understand something well and make it their own when they have learned it from another, compared to when they have learned it for themselves. (Descartes)*

The difference between this module and the previous one is that the instructor performs the technique proficiently from the beginning, washing his hands, wearing a hat, mask, and gloves, etc., up to the fixation of the epidural catheter on the simulator's back. In essence, a before, an after, and a context are added to the pure and simple technique.

The epidural simulator is completed with the addition of all those external elements to the simulator that allow it to reproduce and repropose the development of the real technique (sterile drapes, gloves, hat and mask, local anesthesia, etc.) and accompanied by a trolley on which to arrange the necessary materials for the execution of the technique and the sterile drapes.

In this module, each student performs the complete technique with or without the intervention of the tutor (four-handed technique), depending on the case.

The epidural technique can also be performed with the aid of a checklist.

In this phase, particular attention will be paid to explaining to the students:

1. The methods related to sterility (how to wash hands, how to correctly wear sterile gloves, how to disinfect the skin).
2. How to perform local anesthesia.
3. How to insert the epidural catheter and solve problems related to its insertion.
4. How to aspirate the catheter.
5. How to secure the catheter to the skin and prevent its dislocation.

## 6.1 Sterility of Execution

For training in methods for maintaining sterility, checklists can be used, such as the one described in Table 1 [9].

## 6.2 Local Anesthesia

The teacher must clarify that local anesthesia represents an important moment of the procedure, being both the operator's "business card" and the indispensable condition for proceeding smoothly (both for the patient and the anesthetist) to the technique. The advantages of not abandoning the chosen landmarks for the identification of the interspinous space (the operator's fingers) and proceeding continuously, injecting the anesthetic solution in the ideal direction that will be used to insert the Tuohy needle later [10] will be shown.

**Table 1** Examiner's checklist for aseptic technique. From [9] with permission

| | |
|---|---|
| 1. | Removes rings and watches |
| 2. | Washes hands upon entering the room |
| 3. | Wears a hat and a face mask |
| 4. | Opens the epidural tray in the correct manner and sequence (upper flap opened away from the operator) |
| 5. | Washes hands with alcohol gel and air dries them |
| 6. | Wears gloves in a sterile manner |
| 7. | Prepares the skin aseptically and waits for the solution to dry |
| 8. | Applies the drape in a sterile manner |
| 9. | Works in a way that minimizes the crossing of bare forearms over the sterile field/equipment |
| 10. | Keeps all epidural equipment on the sterile tray when not in use |
| 11. | Maintains control over the catheter tip to avoid contamination |
| 12. | Dries the entry site of the epidural catheter and covers it with a sterile dressing while maintaining sterility (this requires keeping a sterile hand on the catheter insertion site, while partially removing the drape with the other hand to allow the nurse to apply the dressing) |
| 13. | Further removal of any residual antiseptic or blood in the surrounding area is completed only after the entry site itself has been protected by the sterile dressing |

0 = did not perform; 1 = performed inadequately; 2 = performed adequately

## 6.3 Epidural Catheter

As for the epidural catheter, the teacher will remind the students of the characteristics of the type of material in use: the total length and its priming, the fact that the three helical holes are placed in the first centimeter from the closed tip, and the presence of markers indicating the distances from the tip. It will be clarified that the epidural catheter must be inserted inside the epidural space no less than 2 cm and no more than 4 cm to reduce the risk of accidental dislocation or malpositioning in an intervertebral foramen (cause of unilateral analgesia). Together with the students, he will discuss how to insert the catheter deep enough into the tissues to obtain the correct epidural positioning and how it is more logical to insert it deeper than necessary and then withdraw it.

During this session, it is likely that some students will have difficulty introducing the epidural catheter. This is the right time to discuss the diagnosis and resolution of problems related to difficulty in introduction or malpositioning.

## 6.4 Aspiration

Training in catheter aspiration should be done with a small-caliber syringe (2–5 mL to prevent epidural vessels from collapsing) and associated with the observation of any passive reflux (detectable if the catheter is placed lower than the patient's heart). Although the epidural simulator (unless it also provides this function and/or has been previously prepared *ad hoc*) cannot usually realistically mimic blood/cerebrospinal fluid reflux, students should be instructed, trained, and accustomed to performing these two simple safety maneuvers that should certainly be included in the epidural technique checklist. As for the test dose, it represents a topic too complex and extensive to be addressed in this module, so the teacher should plan a separate session entirely dedicated to explaining the theoretical basis of the test dose and prevention techniques for accidental vascular or subarachnoid administration in both cesarean section anesthesia and labor analgesia. In that lesson, the principles of treatment for local anesthetic toxicity can also be presented, with particular reference to pregnancy.

### 6.5 Fixing the Catheter to the Skin

Usually, students do not pay much attention to how to fix the epidural catheter to the skin or get distracted by the many possible fixation variants suggested by different tutors. In addition to expressing their personal opinion, it is appropriate for the teacher to state the theory of good fixation: "the anchoring point of the epidural catheter is the ligamentum flavum, so, in any way you fix it to the skin, it is essential that the anchoring point to the ligamentum flavum offers greater resistance to stretching than the fixation point to the skin you have prepared, otherwise it is likely that the catheter will dislocate from the epidural space during the patient's movements or with the simple passage from the sitting to the supine position."

If a high-fidelity mannequin and a simulation center are not available, this module can include performance evaluations with the checklist and the epidural global rating scale (Chap. "Assessing Learning", Fig. 7) by the teacher and self-assessment by the student (see Chap. "Assessing Learning"). Otherwise, proceed to module 7.

## 7 Module 7: The Technique as in the Real World

*The true truths are those that can be invented. (Kraus)*

This optional module requires a complete simulation room with a high-fidelity mannequin to allow the execution of the technique in a highly realistic environment reproducing the delivery room and/or operating room, with a scenario involving actors (patient, nurse, colleague).

The high-fidelity mannequin is placed in a lateral position with the epidural simulator inserted inside, and the room is prepared *ad hoc* to reproduce and repropose the real technique execution (sterile drapes, gloves, hat and mask, preparation of the trolley, local anesthesia, etc.) and the delivery room environment (ongoing maternal and fetal monitoring).

Each student (dressed as in the operating room) will perform the block starting from the explanation to be given to the patient, after obtaining informed consent and after preparing themselves in a sterile manner to perform the procedure. The

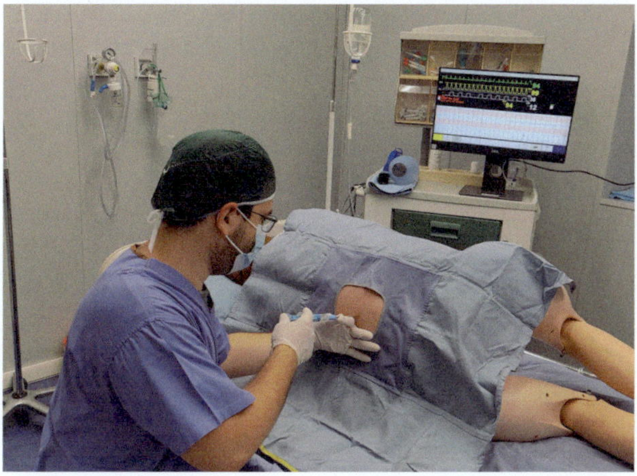

**Fig. 37** The high-fidelity mannequin is placed in a lateral position with the epidural simulator inserted inside, and the simulation room is prepared ad hoc to reproduce and repropose the real technique execution (sterile drapes, gloves, hat and mask, preparation of the trolley, local anesthesia, etc.) and the delivery room environment (ongoing maternal and fetal monitoring)

scenario is prepared so that the mannequin-patient can interact with the student (Fig. 37).

The purpose of the scenario is to have the epidural technique performed in an environment similar to the real one, with active monitoring, the patient interacting, and the delivery room (or operating room) staff who can interfere and/or help the student.

During the scenario, the student can ask for help from the teacher and, at the teacher's discretion, can, if desired, use the checklist as a memo-technique. At the end of the scenario, the teacher will assign a score to the performance using the global assessment rate or a similar scale.

Depending on their skills and the curricular requirements of the school, the teacher can organize a technical and/or behavioral debriefing at the end of the scenario, individually or in the presence of other students who can thus give feedback to their colleague [11].

## 8 Module 8: The Technique on the Patient in Hospital/Operating Room/Labor–Delivery Room

*We do not do anything well until we cease to think about the manner of doing it. (Hazlitt)*

The teaching and practical learning of technical skills to perform an epidural in obstetrics, and especially for labor analgesia, is particularly complex as it involves learning the technique during labor.

If the students have completed the training course described so far and have practiced with the epidural simulator and the simulation scenario, they will be facilitated in learning on the patient, and at the same time, the patient herself will feel more reassured knowing that the doctor in training has already had preliminary training that has certified them.

The subsequent technical steps do not differ much from those already used for learning the technique on the simulator. The four-handed technique previously described will be used.

The tutor and the student should discuss before approaching the patient how to relate during the execution of the block. This is obviously not only for obvious safety reasons, but also to establish in advance, for example, how many attempts the student can make before the tutor intervenes or takes their place and whether this should happen at the student's request or based on the tutor's decision. This joint decision reduces the student's anxiety, especially at the beginning, in case they find themselves or feel without adequate support because the tutor does not actively intervene to help them. It is also appropriate to discuss in advance how to communicate in front of the patient and healthcare personnel. A tool that can be practical is nonverbal communication. For example, a "time out" signal made with the tutor's hands to the student who is struggling and making repeated and unsuccessful attempts to insert the needle can save the patient the discomfort of witnessing the verbal communication between the student and the tutor. It is good practice that whenever possible, the tutor does not comment and discuss technical or behavioral issues with the student in the presence of the patient.

It is usually believed that training in the epidural technique concerns exclusively technical aspects and, subsequently, pharmacological aspects and how to deal with difficult cases or the treatment of any complications. Often the success of the technique also depends on the organizational and interdisciplinary communication skills of the anesthesiologist, so it is essential, from the very first moments of practical training on the patient, that the teacher also takes care of the "relational aspects" of the epidural block, gradually introducing some elements of nontechnical or behavioral skills, for example, how to ask for informed consent for labor analgesia, how to discuss and plan a cesarean section with obstetric colleagues, how to manage the team in the case of complications, how to talk to relatives, etc.

On the real patient, repeating in practice the initial stages previously performed on the simulator, the tutor will initially use the "four-handed" technique (used by the author of this book for 25 years of teaching) (Fig. 38) and then gradually leave full autonomy to the student:

1. Masterful execution by the tutor

   The teacher performs the technique in front of the student according to the rules of the art.

   On this occasion, materials, procedure, and general principles are reviewed.
2. Hands-on execution of the student on the tutor

   The teacher performs the technique, and the student, with sterile gloves, places their hands exactly on those of the tutor, who will communicate aloud all the needle passages in the tissues, relating tactile sensations and anatomical structures crossed.

   It is advisable to perform this technique at least 5–10 times, but not less than 5 times.

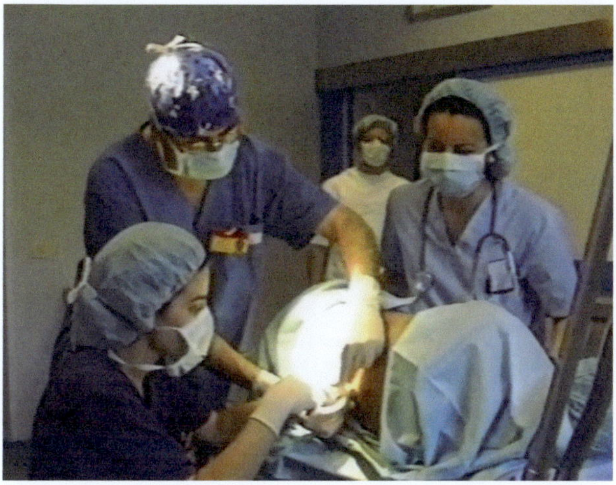

**Fig. 38** The "four-handed" technique performed by the author of this book for 35 years. The photo was taken at the Fatebenefratelli Hospital in Rome in 1986

3. Hands-on execution of the tutor on the student

   The student performs the technique, and the teacher, with sterile gloves, places their hands exactly on those of the student, who will communicate aloud all the steps of the needle through the tissues, relating tactile sensations and anatomical structures crossed. The teacher confirms the student's tactile sensations at each step.

   It is advisable to perform this technique at least 10 times.
4. Student's execution alone with the tutor nearby in the same room

   The student performs the technique completely on their own, but the teacher is beside them.

   Observation and intervention only if requested and necessary.
5. Student's execution alone

   The student performs the technique completely on their own.

   The teacher is not in the same room but is readily available upon request.

## 9 Monitoring and Certification of Students' Skills

The number of epidurals required for the transition to the next step may be varied at the teacher's discretion based on the student's performance and the technical difficulties encountered during training.

A more objective way to decide when the student has reached the necessary competence is to use an individual *CUSUM* curve (see Chap. "Learning Curves"). In this case, the teacher can decide in advance the level of competence that must be reached and monitor its evolution over time based on the type of curve that develops during the training period.

It would be appropriate for each institution to create its own epidural checklist (Fig. 39) or adopt one already in use or certified, in order to standardize the reference standard for all students and to make possible a homogeneous and valid assessment of competence for all.

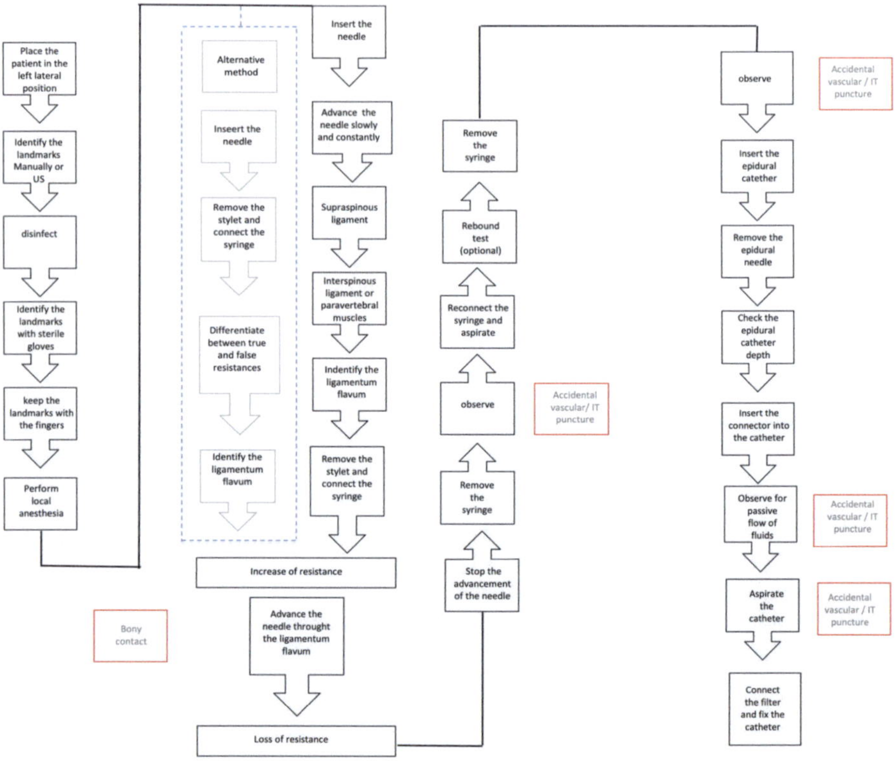


**Fig. 39** The epidural checklist used in our department

Complementary to the checklists are the epidural metrics [12, 13]. We created a set of epidural metrics adapted to our teaching method (Appendix 2).

Metrics are units of observable behavior which together constitute a stepwise description of a reference approach to a procedure, in this case, lumbar epidural block. Assessment outcomes are defined dichotomously as "yes or no" answers depending on whether the defined metric occurred or did not occur. All metrics are defined in terms of errors (deviations from optimal procedure performance).

In order to avoid one of the main limitations of checklists (which is that all phases of the procedural skill considered are weighted equally, regardless of their actual clinical importance), we graded the errors by giving each category a different weight, and eventually, we obtained an overall weighted indicator.

## 10 Conclusions

The structured method not only represents the author's teaching experience in 25 years, but with its most recent modifications (epidural simulator, EMME model, and CompuFlo) constitutes the teaching standard of the European School of

Obstetric Anesthesia (EESOA) in Rome and the source of inspiration for many Italian Universities.

Before being adopted for routine teaching, the model has been validated with a study on trainees. With this structured method, the percentage of residents (who had never performed an epidural block) who reach the necessary competence is doubled compared to their colleagues who are trained in a traditional way [14]. Also, the frequency of accidental dural puncture during the training period in the delivery room is halved.

## Appendix 1: The EMME Model

Eye tracking is a process that monitors eye movements to determine where a subject is looking, what they are looking at, and how long their gaze lingers on a particular point in space.

Eye movement tracking occurs through specific devices that use cameras integrated into glasses that incorporate an infrared system to track the position of the pupil. Detection and interpretation of the associated data are processed through specialized software, using different techniques.

The principle behind the use of eye tracking technology is the theory that suggests a relationship between the point where individuals focus their gaze and the understanding of the cognitive processes that guide this scanning, in essence, what they are paying attention to or thinking about at that moment [15]. The literature has demonstrated the ability of eye tracking to provide reliable quantitative data as an objective assessment tool, with potential applications to medical and surgical training to improve performance [16].

Ocular metrics are able to consistently distinguish nonexperts from experts, and many studies in various medical fields have reported that focused attention and visual representation during the execution of a technical task increase with the improvement of competence for that task [16–19].

This has also been demonstrated for the epidural technique [20], for which different gaze patterns typical of expert anesthetists, who spend more time fixating on a more specific target position, and trainee physicians, who instead divide their attention between monitoring instruments and other different areas and have a more diffuse and less focused gaze (Fig. 40).

Eye tracking, being able to differentiate the visual approach modes of experts from those of beginners, has been employed to evaluate the evolution of skills related to the epidural block of anesthesia residents until the achievement of competence [21].

Recently, eye tracking has been used for the development of new methods to improve teaching and learning processes. The reason is that most information is received through the eyes, and indeed, based on practical experience, we know that simply telling beginners to "watch how the experts do it" in a certain way "works."

Today, it is possible to create task demonstration videos not only by recording an expert's problem-solving behavior and verbal explanations but also by recording

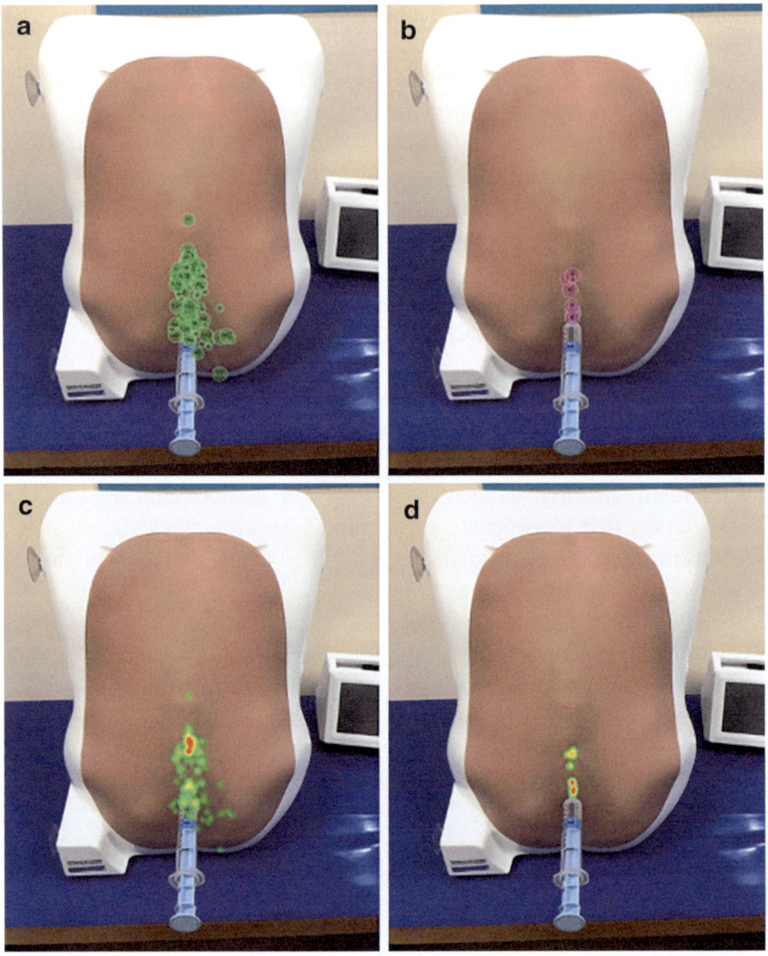


**Fig. 40** Gaze behavior during the execution of epidural block on the epidural simulator. Typical novice's (**a**) and expert's (**b**) gaze plots and novice's (**c**) and expert's (**d**) heatmap. Note the different gaze patterns between experts, who spent more time fixating a more specific target location, and trainees, who split their attention between tracking their tools and other different areas, when performing a simulated epidural technique

and displaying their eye movements overlaid on the information the expert was looking at [22], thus guiding the learner's attention to the information the expert refers to at the right time, thereby promoting their understanding. Video examples with task demonstrations by experts, with the expert's eye movements overlaid on the task, are known as "Eye Movement Modeling Examples" (EMME).

Our group has created an EMME video, using the eye tracking of a group of anesthetists with over 20 years of experience in performing a lumbar epidural block in obstetrics. This video, after being previously validated [23], is currently proposed during teaching module number 5 (Fig. 41).

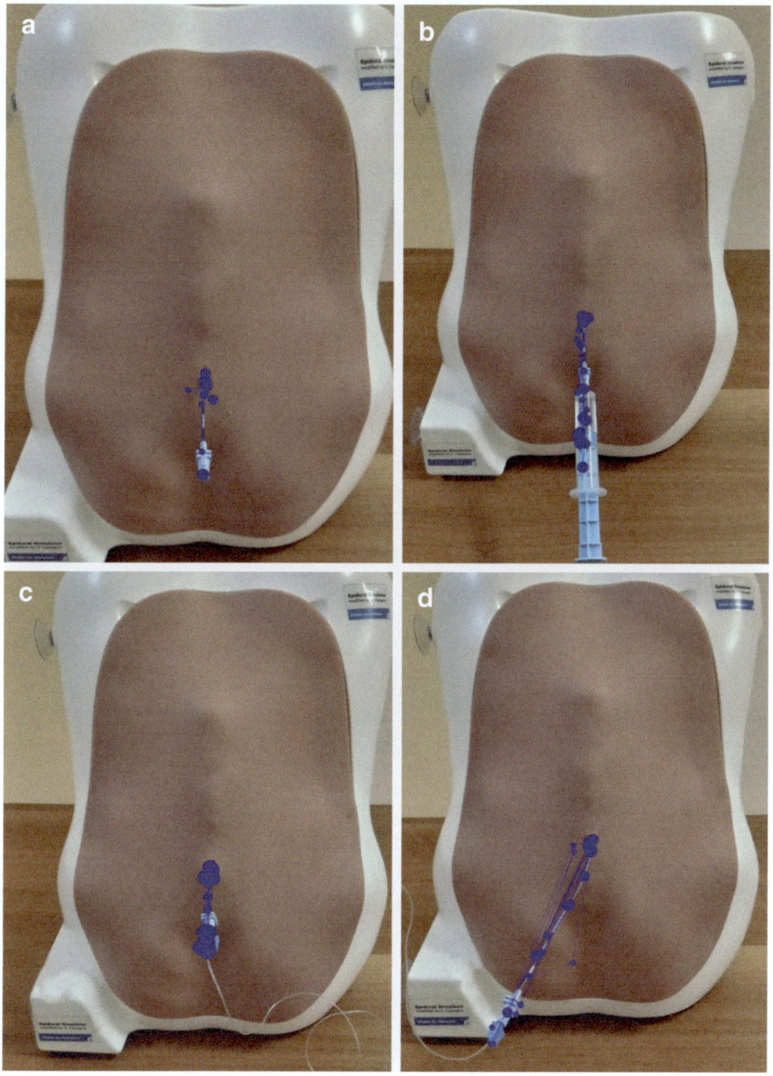

**Fig. 41** Screenshots from the EMME video illustrating where the expert's gaze is focused during the execution of the epidural block: (**a**) during the introduction of the epidural needle; (**b**) during the loss of resistance maneuver; (**c**) during the introduction of the epidural catheter; (**d**) during the removal of the needle

## Appendix 2: Epidural Metrics

I. Placement of the patient (preferably in the lateral position)
1. The patient is not positioned at the edge of the bed.
2. The bed is not flat and parallel to the floor.
3. The patient's head is not flexed on the chest.
4. The patient's legs are not flexed on the abdomen.
5. The patient's shoulders and pelvis are not on the same vertical plane.

II. Identification of the landmarks (manually or by ultrasounds)
6. Tuffier's line is not identified by palpation of the iliac crests.
7. The midline is not appropriately identified through palpation of the spinous processes.
8. US is not used/requested in the case of expected technical difficulty, poor superficial landmarks, or suspected variations in spinal anatomy.

III. Disinfection
9. The trainee does not scrub thoroughly up to the elbow, taking off any rings.
10. Scrubbing not performed in accordance with the guidelines.
11. Asepsis is not maintained during the wearing of sterile gloves.
12. Contaminated drapes are not replaced.
13. Betadine/chlorhexidine solutions contaminate the anesthesia tray/table.
14. In the case of contamination, the trainee does not notice it or/and does not change the contaminated equipment.

IV. Identify the landmarks with sterile gloves
15. The trainee does not request the patient to arch the back.
16. The trainee does not identify landmarks again (palpating iliac crest and/or palpating midline) prior to local infiltration anesthesia.
17. The trainee does not use/request US in the case of expected technical difficulty for poor superficial landmarks or variations in spinal anatomy.

V. Performing local anesthesia
18. The trainee does not warn the patient of the impending puncture.
19. The trainee does not perform a superficial skin wheal.
20. The trainee advances the needle into the tissue quickly and abruptly.
21. The trainee does not gently inject the anesthetic as the needle progresses.
22. The trainee does not allow sufficient time to pass between the injection of the local anesthetic and the insertion of the Tuohy needle (at least 5 s).
23. The trainee uses more than 5 mL of local anesthetic solution for skin infiltration

VI. Inserting the epidural needle
24. The trainee does not hold the needle as he has been taught.
25. The trainee does not warn the patient of the imminent puncture.
26. The trainee does not insert the epidural needle parallel to the chosen interspinous space.

VII. Advancing the needle
 27. The trainee does not advance the needle steadily and very slowly.
 28. The trainee does not stop the needle advancement as soon as she/he feels any increase in resistance.

VIII. Remove the stylet and connect the syringe
 29. Does not hold the Tuohy needle with the back of the nondominant hand on the patient's back.
 30. The stylet of the epidural needle is not placed in the sterile field.
 31. The trainee fills the resistance syringe with more than 5 mL saline.

IX. Differentiate between true and false resistances/identify the ligamentum flavum
 32. The trainee does not recognize the increase in resistance due to the ligamentum flavum (Note 1).
 33. The trainee fails to recognize false loss of resistance (Note 2).
 34. The trainee fails to recognize the true loss of resistance (epidural space) (Note 3).
 35. The trainee fails to recognize or/and is not able to manage the increase in resistance due to bony contact (Note 4).
 36. The trainee fails to recognize/is not able to manage the increase in resistance due to the ligamentum flavum inserted on the vertebral arch (Note 5).

X. Attempts
 37. More than two attempts in the same direction are performed.
 38. No alteration in direction not limited to single plane in any new pass.
 39. Second attempt in the same space without change of angulation in either or both planes.
 40. More than 5 min in the same attempt.

XI. Subsequent attempts
 41. The trainee does not perform a new local anesthesia, if necessary.
 42. The trainee does not prep again if drape is removed.
 43. The trainee undertakes a new attempt in an unprepared and unsterilized interspace.
 44. On seeing blood in the epidural needle, the trainee proceeds with the same needle without flushing with saline or changing the needle.

XII. Checking the needle after loss of resistence
 45. The trainee does not look at the hub of the needle to check for any blood or CSF leaking.
 46. The trainee does not perform a needle aspiration test to check for blood or CSF leaking.

XIII. Catheter insertion
 47. The trainee does not check the depth of the inserted epidural catheter.
 48. The trainee threads the epidural catheter during uterine contractions.
 49. The trainee does not insert the epidural catheter cephalad.
 50. The trainee pulls the catheter back through the needle.
 51. The trainee advances the needle over the catheter at any point.

52. The trainee rotates the epidural needle after the catheter insertion.
53. The trainee inserts the epidural catheter without telling the patient the possibility of having paresthesias.
54. The trainee does not check the epidural catheter depth.
55. The trainee does not place the epidural needle back in the sterile "TRAY."
56. The trainee does not observe the catheter for passive flow of fluids, putting the catheter below the plane of the bed.
57. The trainee does not "gently" aspirate the catheter by using a 2 or 5 mL syringe prior to fixing it or aspirate through the epidural filter.
58. The trainee administers the local anesthetic solution when there is blood in the epidural catheter.
59. If there is blood in the catheter. the trainee does not perform one of the following options: (a) pull back by 1 cm and re-aspirate up to two times, (b) pull catheter out, and (c) flush catheter with saline up to two times.
60. The trainee injects local anesthetic to flush blood out of the epidural catheter.
61. If CSF in the catheter is suspected, the trainee does not perform one of the following actions: (a) Take out the catheter and (b) use it as a spinal catheter.
62. The trainee proceeds to inject local anesthetic dose of >5 mL despite aspirating clear fluid in the epidural catheter.

XIV. Test dose and securing catheter

63. The trainee does not loop the catheter or use a fixating device for taping.
64. The trainee tapes less than halfway up the back.
65. In the case of labor analgesia, more than 10 mL of labor analgesia analgesic solution is used as a test dose or, in the case of cesarean section, more than 3 mL of lidocaine 2%.
66. The trainee administers the test dose during contraction.
67. The trainee does not eventually check for the possible effects of the test dose.

Notes

1. If the needle is inserted into the ligamentum flavum, applying slight pressure on the plunger, the piston does not move because the needle tip is closed by the ligament. By increasing the pressure on the plunger in a continuous, constant, but decisive manner, the needle progresses through the tissues against resistance. Observe that the needle slowly penetrates the tissues while the piston remains stationary.
2. If the needle is *not* inserted into the ligamentum flavum, applying slight pressure on the plunger, the piston moves forward because the needle tip is not closed by the inextensible ligamentum flavum, but by the soft tissues that are easily infiltrated by water.
3. By pushing progressively and constantly on the piston when the needle is in the ligamentum flavum, as soon as the needle tip reaches the epidural space, the

piston is suddenly and unequivocally pushed forward, suddenly discharging the saline solution into the epidural space. Simultaneously, the needle's progression automatically stops.

4. Applying slight pressure on the plunger, the piston moves because the needle tip is against the bone, so resistance can be lost. However, by increasing the pressure on the plunger in a continuous, constant, but decisive manner, the needle does *not* progress through the tissues against resistance. Observe that the needle does *not* slowly penetrate the tissues while the piston remains stationary. Feel the sensation of invincible resistance.
5. Applying slight pressure on the plunger, the piston does not move because the needle tip is inserted into the ligamentum flavum in its portion where it attaches to the bone (vertebral arch). By increasing the pressure on the plunger in a continuous, constant, but decisive manner, the needle does *not* progress through the tissues against resistance. Observe that the needle does *not* slowly penetrate the tissues while the piston remains stationary. Feel the sensation of invincible resistance.

**Item weight**

SEVERE error: an act or attitude that, if not performed or not performed correctly, may directly increase the risk of complications to the patient.

Examples:

- The needle is introduced too quickly and intermittently and uncontrollably, and this may increase the risk of accidental dural puncture.
- Aspiration testing is omitted, increasing the risk of not recognizing an accidental intravascular or subarachnoid injection in advance.

MODERATE error: an act or attitude that, if not performed or not performed correctly, may indirectly increase the risk of complications, or in a direct manner create discomfort for the patient, or in a direct manner create potential prerequisites for the later correction (adjustment) of the procedure.

Examples:

- Inadequate fixation of the epidural catheter to the skin, with the risk of subsequent displacement of the catheter.
- Inadequate local anesthesia, with patient pain upon introduction of the epidural needle and the possible risk of uncontrolled patient movement.

MILD error: all the other cases.

## References


1. Hochman MN, Friedman MJ, Williams W, Hochman C. Interstitial tissue pressure associated with dental injections: a clinical study. Quintessence Int. 2006;37:469–76.
2. Ghelber O, Gebhard RE, Vora S, Hagberg CA, Szmuk P. Identification of the epidural space using pressure measurement with the CompuFlo injection pump—a pilot study. Reg Anesth Pain Med. 2008;33:346–52. https://doi.org/10.1016/j.rapm.2008.01.012.
3. Capogna G, Camorcia M, Coccoluto A, Micaglio M, Velardo M. Experimental validation of the CompuFlo® epidural controlled system to identify the epidural space and its clinical use in difficult obstetric cases. Int J Obstet Anesth. 2018;36:28–33. https://doi.org/10.1016/j.ijoa.2018.04.008. Epub 2018 May 4
4. Gebhard RE, Moeller-Bertram T, Dobecki D, Peralta F, Pivalizza EG, Rupasinghe M, Ilic S, Hochman M. Objective epidural space identification using continuous real-time pressure sensing technology: a randomized controlled comparison with fluoroscopy and traditional loss of resistance. Anesth Analg. 2019;129:1319–27. https://doi.org/10.1213/ANE.0000000000003873.
5. Vaira P, Camorcia M, Palladino T, Velardo M, Capogna G. Differentiating false loss of resistance from true loss of resistance while performing the epidural block with the CompuFlo® epidural instrument. Anesthesiol Res Pract. 2019;2019:5185901. https://doi.org/10.1155/2019/5185901.
6. Ghelber O, Szmuk P, Gebhard R, Katz J, Rabb M, Hagberg C. The Compuflo helps inexperienced operators identify the epidural space in a simulator model. EJA. 2006;23:A 941.
7. Capogna E, Coccoluto A, Gibiino G, Del Vecchio A. Compuflo®-assisted training vs conventional training for the identification of the ligamentum Flavum with an epidural simulator: a brief report. Anesthesiol Res Pract. 2019;2019:3804743. https://doi.org/10.1155/2019/3804743.
8. Friedman Z, Katznelson R, Devito I, Siddiqui M, Chan V. Objective assessment of manual skills and proficiency in performing epidural anesthesia—video-assisted validation. Reg Anesth Pain Med. 2006;31:304–10. https://doi.org/10.1016/j.rapm.2006.04.006.
9. Friedman Z, Siddiqui N, Mahmoud S, Davies S. Video-assisted structured teaching to improve aseptic technique during neuraxial block. Br J Anaesth. 2013;111:483–7. https://doi.org/10.1093/bja/aet062.
10. Capogna G. Epidural technique in obstetric anesthesia. Switzerland: Springer Nature; 2020. p. 72–3.
11. Capogna G, Ingrassia PL, Capogna E, Bernardini M, Valteroni E, Pietrabissa G, Nardone G. Strategic debriefing for advanced simulation. Switzerland: Springer Nature; 2022.
12. Gallagher AG. Metric-based simulation training to proficiency in medical education: what it is and how to do it. Ulster Med J. 2012;81:107–13.
13. Kallidaikurichi Srinivasan K, Gallagher A, O'Brien N, Sudir V, Barrett N, O'Connor R, et al. Proficiency-based progression training: an 'end to end' model for decreasing error applied to achievement of effective epidural analgesia during labour: a randomised control study. BMJ Open. 2018; https://doi.org/10.1136/bmjopen-2017-020099.
14. Scorzoni M, Gonnella GL, Capogna E, Velardo M, Giuri PP, Ciancia M, Capogna G, Draisci G. Achieving lumbar epidural block competency in inexperienced trainees after a structured epidural teaching model: a randomized, single blind, prospective comparison of CUSUM learning curves. Anesthesiol Res Pract. 2022;2022:1738783. https://doi.org/10.1155/2022/1738783.
15. Just MA, Carpenter PA. A theory of Reading: from eye fixations to comprehension. Psychol Rev. 1980;87:329–54. https://doi.org/10.1037/0033-295X.87.4.329.
16. Tien T, Pucher PH, Sodergren MH, Sriskandarajah K, Yang GZ, Darzi A. Eye tracking for skills assessment and training: a systematic review. J Surg Res. 2014;191:169–78. https://doi.org/10.1016/j.jss.2014.04.032.
17. Wilson MR, Vine SJ, Bright E, Masters RS, Defriend D, McGrath JS. Gaze training enhances laparoscopic technical skill acquisition and multi-tasking performance: a randomized, controlled study. Surg Endosc. 2011;25:3731–9. https://doi.org/10.1007/s00464-011-1802-2.

18. Tien T, Pucher PH, Sodergren MH, Sriskandarajah K, Yang GZ, Darzi A. Differences in gaze behaviour of expert and junior surgeons performing open inguinal hernia repair. Surg Endosc. 2015;29:405–13. https://doi.org/10.1007/s00464-014-3683-7.
19. Wilson M, McGrath J, Vine S, Brewer J, Defriend D, Masters R. Psychomotor control in a virtual laparoscopic surgery training environment: gaze control parameters differentiate novices from experts. Surg Endosc. 2010;24:2458–64. https://doi.org/10.1007/s00464-010-0986-1.
20. Capogna E, Salvi F, Delvino L, Di Giacinto A, Velardo M. Novice and expert anesthesiologists' eye-tracking metrics during simulated epidural block: a preliminary, brief observational report. Local Reg Anesth. 2020;13:105–9. https://doi.org/10.2147/LRA.S267879.
21. Capogna E, Salvi F, Del Vecchio A, Velardo M, Capogna G. Changes in gaze behavior during the learning of the epidural technique with a simulator in anesthesia novices. Open J Anesthesiol. 2020;10:361–70. https://doi.org/10.4236/ojanes.2020.1011032.
22. Jarodzka H, Van Gog T, Dorr M, Scheiter K, Gerjets P. Learning to see: guiding students' attention via a Model's eye movements fosters learning. Learn Instr. 2013;25:62–70. https://doi.org/10.1016/j.learninstruc.2012.11.004.
23. Capogna E, Scorzoni M, Gonnella G, Velardo M, Giurì P, Ciancia M, et al. Eye movement modeling examples as a teaching tool for epidural block. Open J Anesthesiol. 2023;13:75–84. https://doi.org/10.4236/ojanes.2023.134007.

# Future Perspectives

Giorgio Capogna

Immersive virtual environments (IVEs), including virtual reality (VR) and augmented reality (AR), have gained immense popularity in medical education healthcare. Using lessons learned from other healthcare specialties and the non-healthcare industry, this chapter describes how IVEs, specifically VR and AR, but also artificial intelligence and metaverse, can enhance medical training and subsequent delivery of patient care within the field of epidural anesthesia.

## 1 Augmented Reality (AR)

Augmented reality is the enrichment of the perception of reality with digital information, not naturally detectable by the five senses. In practice, it is the physical reality we live in, filtered with special effects.

Augmented reality creates an amplified version of reality through the use of digital information, which serves to enhance the real environment. In these cases, the environment is framed through the use of a mobile device camera, such as smartphones and tablets, which creates a base image. Layers of information, such as texts, images, and other multimedia content, are superimposed on this starting image. This construction is called an overlay: the camera reads the object in the frame; the system recognizes it and activates a new layer superimposed and perfectly integrated with reality, enhancing the amount of data related to that object. What is seen, therefore, is an interweaving of real and digital.

Although it is possible to access augmented reality with a smartphone, for greater immersion, specific devices such as glasses that integrate a miniature viewer and a camera are needed. The camera, in addition to taking photos and recording videos,

G. Capogna (✉)
EESOA European School of Obstetric Anesthesia, Rome, Italy
e-mail: capogna.eesoa@gmail.com

© The Author(s), under exclusive license to Springer Nature Switzerland AG 2024

G. Capogna (ed.), *How to Teach the Epidural Block in Obstetric Anesthesia*,
https://doi.org/10.1007/978-3-031-70211-2_7

is used to retrieve information from the real world, so that additional information appears on objects or people displayed.

Augmented reality, therefore, does not serve to lead the person using it into another universe, but enhances the one they are already in, adding interactive content.

One of the first applications of augmented reality technology in anesthesia and perioperative medicine was the identification of anatomical structures for regional blocks and peripheral or central vascular accesses [1].

For example, the AREA (augmented reality system for epidural anesthesia) project [2] developed a new, efficient, and fully automatic algorithm for identifying lumbar levels from panoramic ultrasound images that superimposes the identified ultrasound levels on a live video image of the patient's back. Initially, before needle insertion, a sequence of ultrasound images is acquired from the patient's back, used to generate a panoramic image showing a cross-section of spinal anatomy parallel to the main spinal axis. Subsequently, an automatic image processing technique identifies the lumbar levels in the panoramic image. Finally, an augmented reality module converts the position of the levels in the panoramic image relative to the patient's view from the camera and superimposes virtual markings of the levels on a live video display of the patient's back.

Another study group [3] developed a marker for ultrasound transducers and software for HoloLens, which records the position and triangulation of the ultrasound transducer during preprocedural scans. Once an image of a clear path from the skin to the intrathecal space is acquired, a hologram of the ideal needle path is projected onto the field of view of the anesthetist wearing the HoloLens. The ultrasound probe is removed while the hologram remains in the correct spatial position to display the needle trajectory during the procedure, as if conducting a real-time ultrasound (Fig. 1).

Some researchers [4] have demonstrated that, using an epidural simulator, the use of a portable augmented reality device with superimposed 3D images can facilitate the identification of the epidural space. Both the success rate and accuracy were significantly higher with the use of augmented reality compared to the conventional reference technique with preprocedural CT imaging. In addition, the procedure time was significantly faster with the use of augmented reality compared to the conventional technique (Fig. 2). Currently, augmented reality is used in some centers to assist medical procedures and to improve the accuracy of diagnostics and the quality of surgical interventions, such as the preparation and execution of spinal surgeries [5] or in neurosurgery and neuroscience [6].

This technology, by allowing a complete (rather than two-dimensional) visualization of the patient's anatomy, improves error rates, the speed of interventions, and outcomes (Fig. 3).

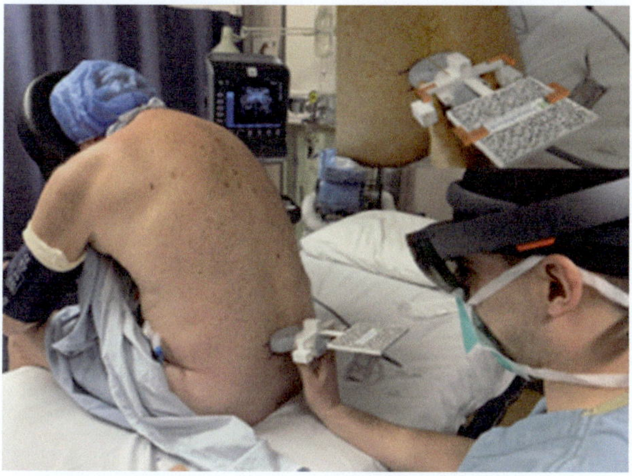

**Fig. 1** The anesthesiologist performs a preprocedural ultrasound, allowing the headset to subsequently generate a spatially stable hologram. The inset shows the operator's mixed reality view displaying a holographic guidance graphic (orange line along the central axis of the ultrasound transducer) with the tracking marker attached to the ultrasound probe. (From [3], an open-access article distributed under the terms of the Creative Commons Attribution License (https://creativecommons.org/licenses/by/4.0/))

## 2 Virtual Reality (VR)

Virtual reality is a technology that leads people into a reality different from the one they live in, existing solely in digital form. It works through the use of devices equipped with sensors, such as gloves and headsets, capable of "transporting" the user into a three-dimensional universe entirely created by a computer, in which they can interact using their body, thus allowing them to recreate and experience any desired experience in the most realistic way possible. In this case, we speak of immersive virtual reality, meaning an environment in which the individual's perception is of being completely isolated from the external environment.

Unlike augmented reality, in which the virtual world "enriches" the real one, in the case of virtual reality, the user immerses themselves in an alternative universe. The main differences between virtual reality and augmented reality are described in Table 1.

Virtual reality has been used therapeutically in anesthesia, as a distractor in the operating room for patients undergoing regional anesthesia, to reduce patient anxiety and increase satisfaction [7], and in the delivery room to reduce pain perception during labor [8].

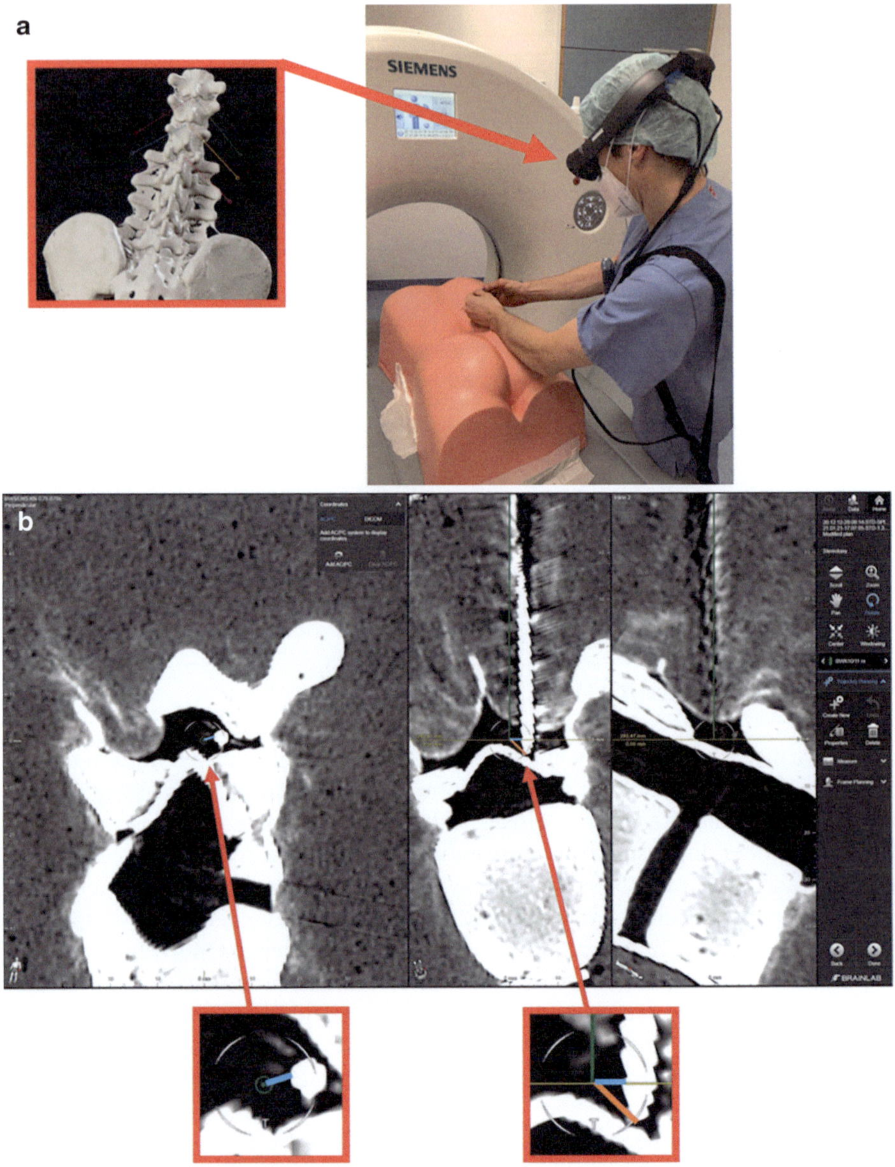


**Fig. 2** Augmented reality-guided puncture of the epidural space and control computed tomography scan. (**a**) Setting for the AR-guided approach with the phantom in prone position and the AR-generated hologram of the spine with trajectories superimposed upon the phantom visible via the AR headset. (**b**) CT scan of the phantom after epidural puncture with the Tuohy needle tip visible in relation to the target point (left panel, green dot) and in relation to the trajectory (right panel, green line). (From [4] with permission)

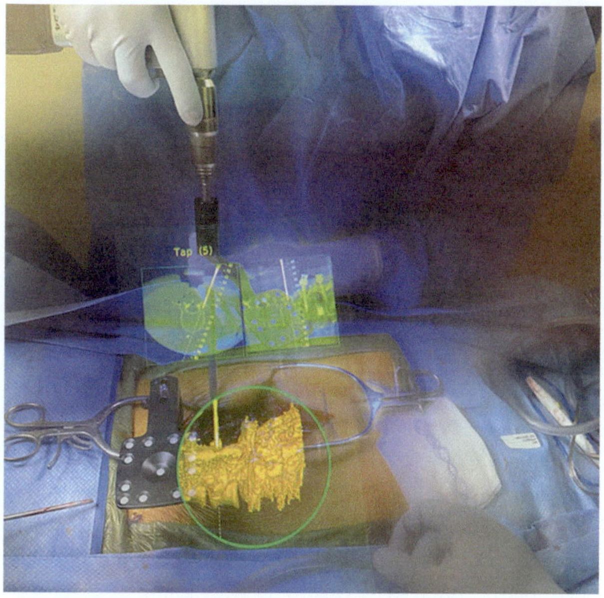


**Fig. 3** Use of augmented reality for a surgical intervention on the spine

**Table 1** Virtual reality and augmented reality: differences and similarities

| Virtual reality | Augmented reality |
|---|---|
| Creates an entire virtual world | Creates a combination of virtual and real world |
| Immersive | Holographic |
| Computer-generated or filmed using 360° camera elements | Computer-generated elements overlaid onto real life |
| Requires a headset | Requires multiple devices |
| Complete immersion in the projected environment using a head-mounted display that completely suppresses the real world (e.g., Google Cardboard and Oculus Rift) | Partial immersion from screen-based devices with cameras (e.g., smartphone, laptop, or tablet) using a head-mounted display with transparent lenses, allowing the viewing of the real world and virtual elements overlaid onto it (e.g., Microsoft HoloLens) |
| Manipulation of objects | Manipulation of objects |
| Only digital objects in the virtual world | Combines physical simulation with virtual objects |

## 3 Artificial Intelligence

Artificial intelligence (AI) is a discipline that studies whether and how intelligent computer systems can be created to simulate human thinking capacity and behavior. Recently, numerous studies have been conducted on the use of artificial intelligence in anesthesiology [9–11].

The more traditional systems of artificial intelligence are those of deductive AI, which are capable of finding patterns in complex streams of existing data, patterns that may be unrecognizable to humans. This can be used to inform decision-making and improve interventions used in clinical practice. The new generative systems, on the other hand, create new data sets inspired by the existing ones. Generative adversarial networks (GANs) are a specific type of machine learning system that has the potential to produce new synthetic data when trained on existing data sets [12]. They work by combining two networks: a generator that learns from an existing data set to produce data and a discriminator that tries to determine whether the data is new or comes from the existing data set. As the system trains, the quality of the data improves. This can be used to create educational material to simulate clinical environments using data in the form of text, video, or images. It is possible to generate case scenarios without worrying about patient data, as the data is simulated. The ability of GANs to produce synthetic data is already widely demonstrated, even in some medical contexts [13].

The potential of AI in monitoring and controlling anesthesia in practice is well documented [14, 15].

In anesthesia and intensive care, as in medicine in general, the use of machine learning would allow each new patient to directly benefit from the data and experience accumulated from treating a large number of previous patients with a similar condition. This experience is accumulated by the system itself in an objective way, and performance will improve with each new patient until the variability of the patient and the procedure are well covered by the data. For anesthesiologists learning to perform a procedure for the first time, this could be particularly important, as the "experience" will be directly accessible through a computer system and not just through lessons taught by expert tutors.

Always in the field of training, AI can implement simulated environments allowing trainees to refine their judgment skills and decision-making processes.

The integration of generative AI systems, such as GANs, with simulations, can create training material more quickly, with more variations and greater fidelity. Given the machine learning nature of generative AI, the systems are intrinsically self-improving. In this way, GANs can be used not only to generate variations on previously written simulations but also to improve them. This is an interesting argument in favor of the development of generative AI systems for training purposes.

## 4 Metaverse

The term "metaverse" was first used in 1992 in the science fiction novel *Snow Crash* by Neal Stephenson [16] to describe a virtual space parallel to the real world. The main body of the space was a virtual city, presented as a featureless black planet. Users could enter the planet from the real world to interact with other users by purchasing virtual land properties and developing buildings on them through virtual reality technology, such as VR glasses and other devices.

With the development and progress of technology, the concept of the metaverse has gradually transformed from virtual to real, and in a broader and more general sense, the metaverse can be defined as a 3D online virtual environment that uses network technology and requires users to access it through VR glasses, mobile phones, computers, and other real-world devices. With the support of communication networks and embedded reality technology, the metaverse realizes the connection between the virtual and real worlds, representing the evolution of the Internet without replacing it.

Currently, the metaverse can be considered an Internet in its infancy: it constitutes the foundations of a new form of communication, without it being clear yet what will be built on top of it and what it will be exactly. In fact, it can be thought of as a set of technologies on which solutions will be based. Just as the Internet is the technology on which email, websites, chat, and streaming are based, so the metaverse is a technology on which a series of applications will be implemented, which for now are still difficult to predict.

The metaverse is a digital universe made up of multiple technological elements, including video, virtual reality, and augmented reality. In the metaverse, users access through 3D viewers and live virtual experiences: they can create realistic avatars, meet other users, create virtual objects or properties, attend concerts, conferences, travel, and more.

Although the metaverse is still in the early stages of development, most healthcare sectors are already hypothesizing and experimenting with its impact.

Many technologies used in the metaverse could have real uses in today's healthcare: augmented reality, virtual reality, and mixed reality, or AR, VR, and MR, collectively referred to as XR; Web3 technologies and applications, such as blockchain and virtual assets; and M-worlds, the "living" virtual places where users gather and create content. So far, most use cases in healthcare involve XR. These technologies are used in various diagnostic and therapeutic applications, as well as in medical training and meetings and conferences. Companies are also experimenting with blockchain for applications ranging from supply chain verification to the storage and management of health data [17].

An in-depth analysis of the potential of the metaverse in medicine has been done by hypothesizing a "CardioVerse" [18], analyzing the infinite possibilities and challenges it entails, introducing new dimensions in education, prevention, and diagnosis of cardiovascular diseases. Its potential applications would be numerous, particularly from improving medical visits and assisting in cardiovascular interventions to reshaping the way medical education is provided. Although the authors foresee obstacles in various areas, such as security, technical, legislative, and regulatory, they suggest, as a potential solution, the use of nonfungible tokens as a security resource for patient data.

## 5 Educational Perspectives

In the immediate future, a rapid expansion of applications in the educational field of virtual reality and augmented reality is expected. The latter, in particular, has a growing demand and can be applied more regularly due to its ability to embrace the surrounding reality, but above all because it has significantly lower development costs compared to virtual reality. Virtual reality, however, has the advantage of allowing students to have real experiences in a digital reality, bridging the gap between a physical and a virtual experience.

## 5.1 Anesthesiology Training Based on Immersive Virtual Environments

Anesthesiology training based on immersive virtual environments (IVE), including virtual reality (VR) and augmented reality (AR), has been reported for procedural areas such as bronchoscopy, insertion of central lines, and epidural haptic simulators [19–22].

Studies that have examined this type of procedural training have shown that practicing technical skills in virtual environments can lead to the effective acquisition and retention of knowledge with subsequent successful clinical application [23, 24].

Furthermore, IVEs can be easily manipulated, allowing for the iterative construction of skills within evolving virtual scenarios. The learning curve may improve because scenarios can change, as they do in the real world.

IVEs can also have significant potential in teaching and assessing nontechnical skills, such as empathy, communication, and decision-making. For example, to address the issue of increasingly crowded clinical environments, reduced working hours for trainees, and pandemic-related restrictions, the use of VR-360 fish-eye video has been proposed to integrate observational learning [25].

This technology has been used to broadcast live surgical interventions to trainees when they are not present in the operating room. VR-360 cameras indeed allow learners to feel as if they were physically present in the learning environment.

Another educational tool is fully immersive computer-generated video game software that mimics clinical environments that can be used to teach both technical skills and decision-making processes related to uncommon crisis situations, such as operating room fires and malignant hyperthermia, or more common scenarios, such as trauma management, anaphylaxis, and obstetric emergencies [26]. In these virtual environments, scenarios can change rapidly and adapt to the needs of learners or specific objectives. Virtual patients improve or worsen in real time, depending on the actions taken by the students. Like in a video game, learners can "restart" and manage crises repeatedly, thanks to the feedback processes integrated into the software. Moreover, these scenarios can be recorded for future viewing or even observed live by a facilitator to provide remote coaching or assessment.

In the field of teaching epidural block, a virtual tutor instructor for epidural block has been created [27]. The authors of this project have created a virtual reality epidural tutor (EET) that can illustrate the epidural by speaking with a synthesized voice. The tutor is connected to a haptic simulator that allows positioning and angling the needle so that each layer of tissue being crossed can be perceived. As soon as the needle is placed inside the simulator, the learner can obtain scores related to needle positioning, catheter insertion, and any injury caused by incorrect needle guidance. The score takes into account the time taken, the number of redirections, the speed of advancement through the layers, the distance traveled by the needle in the epidural space before stopping, and any injuries or pain caused by bone contacts or accidental dural punctures. In addition, if a dural puncture has occurred, it indicates the severity of the injury based on the depth of the perforation.

Within the epidural simulator, a series of tasks and objectives are programmed as described in Table 2. The virtual reality tutor guides the trainee through each task, one by one, until the completion of the epidural or its failure. At the end of the process, a global evaluation card is displayed.

The system also displays the pressure chart during needle insertion, measured by a wireless device placed on the syringe piston, which shows the pressure applied to

**Table 2** Series of assigned tasks to perform and evaluation by the virtual epidural tutor. From [27], with permission

| | Task | Evaluation |
|---|---|---|
| 01 | Palpate the lumbar back and mark the insertion point on the skin | The mark must be clearly visible and not too close to the lamina. Central to the midline or lateral to the paramedian line. Between L2/L3 and L3/L4 |
| 02 | Insert the Tuohy needle through the skin and stop in the subcutaneous fat layer | The needle must not go deeper than the beginning of the supraspinous ligament. The vertical angle must be between 0° and 30°. The horizontal angle must be between 0° and 30°. The needle bevel must face upwards |
| 03 | Fill the syringe with saline solution or air and connect it to the needle. Apply pressure on the plunger to check for the absence of leaks | No air bubbles in the saline solution. The pressure must be between 50 and 500 mmHg |
| 04 | Slowly, applying intermittent or continuous pressure on the plunger, use force on the wings of the Tuohy needle to penetrate through the supraspinous and interspinous ligaments until reaching the ligamentum flavum | The pressure must be between 50 and 500 mmHg. The needle must stop before piercing the ligamentum flavum. If operation 04 is incomplete due to contact with bone, proceed to operation 07 |
| 05 | Cross the ligamentum flavum and immediately stop the needle to avoid going further | The pressure must suddenly decrease at the point of loss of resistance. The needle must pass through the ligamentum flavum. The dura must not be pierced |
| 06 | Once the epidural space is found, remove the syringe and place the catheter | The needle must be removed while the catheter remains in situ. The dura must not be pierced |
| 07 | After encountering bone, withdraw the needle to the fat layer, reattach the syringe, and continue from task 04 | The pressure must suddenly decrease at the point of loss of resistance. The needle must pass through the ligamentum flavum. The dura must not be pierced. Training completed |
| 08 | In the case of accidental dural puncture, stop the epidural, carefully withdraw the needle completely, and perform a blood patch | Correct application of blood patch without injuries |

the physiological solution during insertion. The system allows users to view the pressure chart in real time during insertion and could help them develop the epidural technique so that it matches the execution modes of experts.

The tasks assigned by the virtual tutor include the main aspects that must be learned for epidural training. The system seems to provide a method for objectively assessing the learning of the epidural procedure in a fair way for all trainees, providing constructive feedback that can help identify areas of the technique that need further work.

### 5.2 Potential Use of the Metaverse

The potential use of the metaverse has been hypothesized in many medical specialties, such as cardiology [18], psychiatry [28], dentistry [29], and obstetrics and gynecology [30].

The potential implications of the metaverse in healthcare are far-reaching. By leveraging virtual reality and augmented reality technology, healthcare professionals could be able to provide more accurate diagnoses, treatments, and surgical interventions than ever before.

With the introduction of the metaverse, healthcare could become more efficient, personalized, and cost-effective. Virtual health visits, remote surgical simulations, real-time patient monitoring, and remote robotic surgeries could become possible. This could dramatically reduce healthcare costs while improving the quality of care.

The most obvious implication of the metaverse in healthcare is the possibility of performing remote surgeries, which could be conducted with a much higher degree of accuracy and precision than in the past. Augmented reality could be used to streamline and optimize surgical procedures, allowing surgeons to view 3D images of organs and tissues in real time. By creating a digital twin of the patient's body, doctors would be able to have a detailed view of the patient's anatomy without having to open them up for surgery.

The potential implications of the metaverse in healthcare are virtually limitless, as could be the educational ones aimed at young doctors in training.

It is difficult, given the current state of knowledge, to predict the role that emerging and future technologies will have on educational processes in healthcare.

## 6 Conclusions

The training path of a person, and therefore also of our anesthesiology students, is the link that binds generations together, building on the transmission of knowledge. Due to the speed of technological changes at our disposal, we have already witnessed the loss of "know-how"; with the introduction of artificial intelligence, we could witness the loss of "knowing how to think." The acceleration of communication and information makes it difficult for our brain to acquire culture through sedimentation. The past, traditional one-to-one teaching, and the teacher–student relationship could become obsolete or useless when everything changes quickly and is always available, currently on the Internet, in the future in the metaverse and through artificial intelligence. The challenge of the future will be to redesign training paths, knowing how to use the new while respecting the past and the present because knowledge is a continuous construction process that involves not only the rational but also the consciousness and emotions of human beings. As for the use of artificial intelligence in teaching, it is still too early to predict its role. However, it should be noted that the leaders of the main artificial intelligence companies have sounded an alarm that the technology they are building should be considered a risk to society on a par with "pandemics and nuclear wars," in a document from the Center for AI Safety (https://www.safe.ai/work-summary) signed by executives, researchers, and engineers in this field, raising concerns that AI could soon be used on a global scale to spread disinformation and propaganda, or that it could eliminate millions of jobs if nothing is done to slow it down or regulate it adequately and rigorously.

## References


1. Privorotskiy A, Garcia VA, Babbitt LE, Choi JE, Cata JP. Augmented reality in anesthesia, pain medicine and critical care: a narrative review. J Clin Monit Comput. 2022;36:33–9. https://doi.org/10.1007/s10877-021-00705-0.
2. Al-Deen Ashab H, Lessoway VA, Khallaghi S, Cheng A, Rohling R, Abolmaesumi P. An augmented reality system for epidural anesthesia (AREA): prepuncture identification of vertebrae. IEEE Trans Biomed Eng. 2013;60:2636–44. https://doi.org/10.1109/TBME.2013.2262279.
3. Tanwani J, Alam F, Matava C, Choi S, McHardy P, Singer O, Cheong G, Wiegelmann J. Development of a head-mounted holographic needle guidance system for enhanced ultrasound-guided Neuraxial anesthesia: system development and observational evaluation. JMIR Form Res. 2022;6:e36931. https://doi.org/10.2196/36931.
4. Reinacher PC, Cimniak A, Demerath T, Schallner N. Usage of augmented reality for interventional neuraxial procedures: a phantom-based study. Eur J Anaesthesiol. 2023;40:121–9. https://doi.org/10.1097/EJA.0000000000001755.
5. Dibble CF, Molina CA. Device profile of the XVision-spine (XVS) augmented-reality surgical navigation system: overview of its safety and efficacy. Expert Rev Med Devices. 2021;18:1–8. https://doi.org/10.1080/17434440.2021.1865795.
6. Scott H, Griffin C, Coggins W, Elberson B, Addeldayem M, Virmani TT, et al. Virtual reality in the neurosciences: current practice and future directions. Front Surg. 2022;8:1–13. https://doi.org/10.3389/fsurg.2021.807195.
7. Alaterre C, Duceau B, Sung Tsai E, Zriouel S, Bonnet F, Lescot T, Verdonk F. Virtual reality for peripheral regional anesthesia (VR-PERLA study). J Clin Med. 2020;13(9):215. https://doi.org/10.3390/jcm9010215.
8. Wong MS, Spiegel BMR, Gregory KD. Virtual reality reduces pain in laboring women: a randomized controlled trial. Am J Perinatol. 2021;38:e167–72. https://doi.org/10.1055/s-0040-1708851.
9. Char DS, Burgart A. Machine-learning implementation in clinical anesthesia: opportunities and challenges. Anesth Analg. 2020;130:1709–12. https://doi.org/10.1213/ANE.0000000000004656.
10. Connor CW. Artificial intelligence and machine learning in anesthesiology. Anesthesiology. 2019;131:1346–59. https://doi.org/10.1097/ALN.0000000000002694.

11. Shorten G, Srinivasan KK, Reinertsen I. Machine learning and evidence-based training in technical skills. Br J Anaesth. 2018;121:521–3. https://doi.org/10.1016/j.bja.2018.04.012.
12. Kazuhiro K, Werner RA, Toriumi F, Javadi MS, Pomper MG, Solnes LB, Verde F, Higuchi T, Rowe SP. Generative adversarial networks for the creation of realistic artificial brain magnetic resonance images. Tomography. 2018;4:159–63. https://doi.org/10.18383/j.tom.2018.00042.
13. Fujioka T, Mori M, Kubota K, Kikuchi Y, Katsuta L, Adachi M, et al. Breast ultrasound image synthesis using deep convolutional generative adversarial networks. Diagnostics. 2019;9:176. https://doi.org/10.3390/diagnostics9040176.
14. Hashimoto DA, Witkowski E, Gao L, Meireles O, Rosman G. Artificial intelligence in anesthesiology: current techniques, clinical applications, and limitations. Anesthesiology. 2020;132:379–94. https://doi.org/10.1097/ALN.0000000000002960.
15. Bellini V, Valente M, Bertorelli G, Pifferi B, Craca M, Mordonini M, et al. Machine learning in perioperative medicine: a systematic review. J Anesth Analg Crit Care. 2022;2:2. https://doi.org/10.1186/s44158-022-00033-y.
16. Stephenson N. Snow crash. New York: Bantam Books; 1992.
17. Lee CW. Application of Metaverse service to healthcare industry: a strategic perspective. Int J Environ Res Public Health. 2022;19:13038. https://doi.org/10.3390/ijerph192013038.
18. Skaldis I, Muller O, Fournier S. CardoVerse: the cardiovascular medicine in the era of Metaverse. Trends Cardiovasc Med. 2022.; in press; https://doi.org/10.1016/j.tcm.2022.05.004.
19. Casso G, Schoettker P, Savoldelli GL, Azzola A, Cassina T. Development and initial evaluation of a novel, ultraportable, virtual reality bronchoscopy simulator: the computer airway simulation system. Anesth Analg. 2019;129:8–8.
20. Moo-Young J, Weber TM, Kapralos B, Quevedo A, Alam F. Development of unity simulator for epidural insertion training for replacing current lumbar puncture simulators. Cureus. 2021;13:8.
21. Huang VW, Jones CB, Gomez ED. State of the art of virtual reality simulation in anesthesia. Int Anesthesiol Clin. 2020;58:8–8.
22. Barrie M, Socha JJ, Mansour L, Patterson ES. Mixed reality in medical education: a narrative literature review. Proc Int Symp Hum Factors Ergon Health Care. 2019;8:88.
23. Mao RQ, Lan L, Kay J, Lohre R, Ayeni OR, Goel DP, et al. Immersive virtual reality for surgical training: a systematic review. J Surg Res. 2021;268:40–58. https://doi.org/10.1016/j.jss.2021.06.045.
24. Chen S, Zhu J, Cheng C, Pan Z, Liu L, Du J, et al. Can virtual reality improve traditional anatomy education programmes? A mixed-methods study on the use of a 3D skull model. BMC Med Educ. 2020;20:395. https://doi.org/10.1186/s12909-020-02255-6.
25. Blair C, Walsh C, Best P. Immersive 360° videos in health and social care education: a scoping review. BMC Med Educ. 2021;21:590. https://doi.org/10.1186/s12909-021-03013-y.
26. Kononowicz AA, Woodham LA, Edelbring S, Stathakarou N, Davies D, Saxena N, et al. Virtual patient simulations in health professions education: systematic review and meta-analysis by the digital health education collaboration. J Med Internet Res. 2019;21:e14676. https://doi.org/10.2196/14676.
27. Vaughan N, Dubey VN, Wee MYK, Isaacs R. Virtual reality simulation based assessment objectives for epidural training. ASME J Med Devices. 2014;8(2):020948. https://doi.org/10.1115/1.4027064.
28. Shu S, Woo BKP. Pioneering the metaverse: the role of the metaverse in an aging population. JMIR Aging. 2023;6:e40582. https://doi.org/10.2196/40582.30.
29. Kurian N, Cherian JM, Varghese KG. Dentistry in the metaverse. Br Dent J. 2022;232:191. https://doi.org/10.1038/s41415-022-4003-6.
30. Werner H, Ribeiro G, Arcoverde V, Lopes J, Velho L. The use of metaverse in fetal medicine and gynecology. Eur J Radiol. 2022;150:110241. https://doi.org/10.1016/j.ejrad.2022.110241.

MIX
Papier aus verantwortungsvollen Quellen
Paper from responsible sources
FSC® C105338

If you have any concerns about our products,
you can contact us on
**ProductSafety@springernature.com**

In case Publisher is established outside the EU,
the EU authorized representative is:
**Springer Nature Customer Service Center GmbH**
**Europaplatz 3, 69115 Heidelberg, Germany**

Printed by Libri Plureos GmbH
in Hamburg, Germany